NATURE'S
Miracle
MEDICINES

Amazing Remedies from Mother Earth

JEFFREY LAIGN
CONSULTANTS: SILENA HERON, N.D.
& ERIC YARNELL, N.D.

PUBLICATIONS INTERNATIONAL, LTD.

Jeffrey Laign is a writer and editor with a special involvement in herbs and natural healing. An author of many magazine articles and books, including *The Complete Book of Herbs*, he has also been managing editor for Health Communications, Inc.

Dr. Silena Heron is a naturopathic physician with a family health-care practice. She is a nationally recognized specialist in botanical medicine who has taught throughout the West and Canada since 1973. She was founding chair of botanical medicine at Bastyr University and on the faculty for six years. Currently, she is an adjunct faculty member at Southwest College of Naturopathic Medicine. Dr. Heron is technical consultant to a botanical pharmaceutical company and consultant for the publication *The Healing Garden*. She is also the founding vice president of the Botanical Medicine Academy, an accrediting organization for the clinical use of herbal medicines.

Dr. Eric Yarnell is a naturopathic physician, author, editor, and lecturer. He serves as research editor for the *Journal of Naturopathic Medicine* and teaches at the Southwest College of Naturopathic Medicine. He is co-author of *The Phytotherapy Research Compendium*, contributor to *The Natural Pharmacy*, and consultant on *The Healing Garden*. Dr. Yarnell helped found and is currently treasurer of the Botanical Medicine Academy.

Picture credits:

Front cover (inset) and interior illustrations: **Marlene Donnelly; Jean Emmons.**

FPG International: Jeff Baker: 154; Ed Braverman: 59; Mark Harmel: 102, 222; Dick Luria: 100; Jose Luis Banus-March: 85; Art Montes De Oca: 122; R. Pleasant: 39; Telegraph Colour Library: 9, 185; **International Stock:** Scott Barrow: 148, 172, 226; Clint Clemens: 238; Earl Kogler: 175; Jeff Noble: 33; Patrick Ramsey: 193; **Coco McCoy/Rainbow:** 46; **SuperStock:** 69, 81, 114, 128, 143, 203, 206, 237.

CONTENTS

INTRODUCTION

From the dawn of human history, nature has supplied us with both food and medicine. By observing the behavior of animals, early humans learned through trial and error which plants were safe and nutritious to eat and which would be harmful. Animals no doubt also taught ancient men and women that certain plants have healing properties, but others should be shunned as poisons.

The knowledge our ancestors gained has been passed down for centuries. And it has served humankind well.

But as human civilization developed, and as nations became industrialized, our focus shifted to the fruits of our own creations. We turned to laboratories, and the chemicals and machines we learned to create, to provide us with medicine and even "new and improved" food.

With the development of antibiotics in the 1930s, many of us became convinced that we could create all the medicines we would ever need to fight the infections and diseases that threatened to do us in. And, indeed, modern medicine has worked what at one time would have been deemed miracles. Many of the infections and diseases that used to kill millions of all ages have been eradicated or brought under control through the advances of medicine.

Of late, however, we have begun to see some of the down sides and gaps in modern medicine. We have overused antibiotics to the point that some strains of bacteria are no longer killed off by them. And many of the pills we have grown accustomed to popping to ease aches, pains, and other discomforts have turned out to have unpleasant, and at times dangerous, side effects.

The result has been a growing interest in rediscovering the remedies that nature has always provided. We have turned an eye toward the seeming miracles that nature, too, can perform.

In this book, we explore some of the most promising of nature's medicines—those that seem to work *with* rather than against our bodies to ease what ails us. And we investigate natural remedies that appear to fill gaps in modern medicine's arsenal. For example, you'll read of the research supporting the use of the herb echinacea. This plant may bring relief from colds and flu—relief that pharmaceuticals have yet to adequately supply. And unlike the pharmaceuticals that *are* available, echinacea appears to enhance the body's ability to heal itself rather than merely stifling the very symptoms that serve as the body's defenses.

Can natural remedies cure all things that ail us? Not likely. Are herbs and other natural substances safe and effective in every case? No. Should you blindly "pop" herbs the way some of us might pop pills? Definitely not.

Like all things, even the water and oxygen we require for life, natural remedies can be harmful as well as beneficial. Fortunately, most tend to be milder than pharmaceuticals and appear to be less likely to cause harm. But since they are not regulated the way drugs are, the processed herbs that are available in stores may not always contain enough of the ingredients that provide healing. Trial and error appears to once again be in order.

Research has been giving us more and more reasons to continue to explore nature's healing potential. Is that reason to totally abandon modern medical care? Absolutely not. Modern medicine can help us to prevent many diseases and treat a vast array as well. The more prudent approach would be to complement modern medicine's benefits with those that nature can provide.

Read the information in this book. Discuss it with a health care practitioner who likewise sees the wisdom of combining the best of both worlds. Together, you can experiment to find the remedies that work best for your body. And together, you may realize the miracle of healing.

ST. JOHN'S WORT FOR DEPRESSION

St. John's wort was used by ancient Greek physicians to treat wounds. In the Middle Ages, it was said to ward off evil spirits. Today, many researchers are hopeful that the ubiquitous weed may hold the key to safely and effectively fighting the demon of depression, the most common mental health problem of our angst-ridden culture. Consumers as well are discovering the benefits of St. John's wort, judging by sales figures at health-food stores and drugstores around the country.

Because its yellow flowers produce a bright red oil when crushed, bygone healers (as well as folk healers today) used St. John's wort primarily to treat blood-related conditions, such as wounds. They also used it for infections, menstrual problems, anxiety, and depression. Now scientists are beginning to confirm that St. John's wort's greatest contribution may indeed be as a natural antidepressant. In clinical trial after clinical trial, St. John's wort extracts have successfully alleviated symptoms of mild to moderate depression without causing many of the unpleasant, often dangerous, side effects produced by synthetic drugs.

What Is Depression?

Most people feel "down" or "blue" once in a while. But depression is more than that. It is a medical disorder that affects your thoughts, feelings, behavior, and physical health.

People who suffer from depression have a number of symptoms nearly every day, all day, for at least two weeks. Symptoms of depression include:

- feelings of sadness, hopelessness, helplessness, and irritability

- withdrawal from human contact

- change in appetite, weight loss when not dieting, or weight gain

- change in sleep habits, fitful sleep, inability to fall asleep, or sleeping too much

- loss of interest in activities formerly enjoyed

- inability to concentrate or make decisions

- feelings of worthlessness

- inappropriate feelings of guilt

- fatigue
- recurring thoughts of death or suicide or attempting suicide (This symptom requires immediate medical attention.)

Many depressed people have mental and physical symptoms that seem endless and do not get better with happy events or good news. Some depressed people are so disabled by their condition that they don't even have enough energy to call a friend, relative, or medical professional for help.

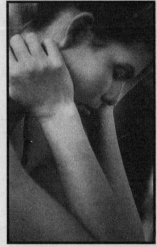

Depression is the most common psychological

Depression can cause an overwhelming feeling of sadness.

problem in the United States, plaguing more than 17 million people a year at a cost of $44 billion, including $24.2 billion for lowered productivity and job absenteeism and $12.3 billion for medical and psychiatric care.

Anyone can get depressed. It's an equal-opportunity illness, striking all races and people in every socioeconomic group. Depression occurs at all ages, although major depressive episodes peak between the ages of 55 and 70 in men and 20 and 45 in women. The illness in some form affects 25 percent of women, 10 percent of men, and 5 percent of adolescents worldwide.

About half of those who have an episode of major depression will have another within two years. For some people, episodes of depression are separated by several years, while other people suffer a series of episodes in a short time. Between episodes, such individuals feel well.

What Causes Depression?

Depression may be related to many factors, including a family history of depression, medical illnesses, alcohol, drugs (even some prescription medications), gender, and age. Additionally, a person's self-confidence, personality traits (such as dependency on others or perfectionism), and unrealistic expectations may lead to depression. Stressful events, such as the death of a spouse or loss of a job, also contribute.

There are many theories about the causes of depression. The social-learning theory suggests that lack of positive reinforcement from others may lead to negative self-evaluation and a poor outlook on the future. The psychoanalytic theory suggests that a significant loss (such as of a parent) or a withdrawal of affection in childhood (whether real or perceived) may lead to depression later in life. Interpersonal theory emphasizes the importance of social connections for good mental health. Other theories suggest that unrealistic expectations of oneself and others and loss of self-esteem are essential contributors to depression.

Some individuals may be biologically predisposed to depression; in other words, they may have been born with a tendency to develop depression. Depression often runs in families. For example, if one identical twin suffers from depression or manic-depression (a type of depression marked by episodes of mania followed by depression), the other twin has a 70 percent chance of also having the illness.

Research indicates that some people suffering from depression have imbalances in neurotransmitters (chemical messengers that relay signals between nerve cells) in the brain. The neurotransmitters that are often out of balance in depressed people are serotonin, norepinephrine, and dopamine. Several neurotransmitter imbalances may be involved; researchers are seeking other neurotransmitters that may also play a role in depression.

In general, researchers view depression as the result of interaction between environmental and biological factors. Depression may be endogenous (internally caused) or exogenous (related to outside events). Major changes in one's environment, such as a move or job change, or any major loss, such as a divorce or the death of a loved one, can bring on depression. Feeling depressed in response to these changes is normal, but when it becomes a severe long-term condition (longer than one month) and interferes with effective functioning, it requires treatment.

Some environmental factors relating to depression include being unemployed, poor, elderly, or alone. Depression changes one's way of looking at ordinary life circumstances. A depressed person tends to exaggerate negative aspects, which leads to feelings of hopelessness, helplessness, and being overwhelmed.

St. John's Wort at a Glance

Latin name: *Hypericum*

Description: St. John's wort actually refers to about 200 species within the genus *Hypericum*, of the Hypericaceae family. The species used in the treatment of depression is *Hypericum perforatum (H. perforatum)*, and it is the *Hypericum* referred to throughout this chapter. A hardy perennial,

Debilitating diseases can severely restrict one's usual lifestyle, resulting in depression. Illnesses that affect brain functioning and impair blood flow to the brain can produce depression. Such illnesses may include malfunctions of the thyroid or parathyroid gland, diseases that affect the nerves, nutritional disorders, and infectious diseases. Depression can also occur as a side effect of certain medications (see page 19).

Women, moreover, seem to suffer more from depression than do men. Some researchers argue that this disparity is caused by hormonal differences; others suggest that the difference results from socialization. Girls in western society are taught to monitor their feelings and to ask for help when they are troubled. Boys, on the other hand, are encouraged to ignore their feelings and handle problems on their own. Thus, it may be that men and women are equally likely to be-

H. perforatum is an erect plant with small, oblong, light green leaves and five-petalled, bright yellow flowers, which bloom from late June through August. If you pinch or crush the flowers, they turn red. St. John's wort has a characteristic smell, something like balsam.

Habitat: Brought over from Europe, St. John's wort has become naturalized throughout the United States and may be found as a roadside weed or in woods and meadows.

come depressed, but that men are more reluctant to admit that they are feeling down.

The Ups and Downs of Antidepressants

Until fairly recently, there wasn't much doctors could do to treat depression, beyond listening and talking to their patients. Psychotherapy still plays a vital role in treating depression. But the discovery of pharmaceutical antidepressants in the 1950s was heralded as a major medical breakthrough.

The first drug found to help depressed people actually started out as a potential treatment for tuberculosis (TB). Drug researchers discovered that the drug, iproniazid (Marsilid), tended to lift the TB patients' mood. So, in 1952, the drug was introduced as a treatment for depression. Iproniazid and subsequent drugs like it fall into a class of drugs called monoamine oxidase (MAO) inhibitors, which work by reducing the quantity of the enzyme monoamine oxidase. Monoamine oxidase breaks down excess amines (such as norepinephrine, serotonin, and dopamine) in the brain. By inhibiting monoamine oxidase, more of these amines remain in the brain, which in turn reduces the symptoms of depression. The MAO inhibitors fell out of favor in the early 1960s when scientists realized they could cause a deadly reaction when taken with foods that contain a substance called tyramine (see page 17). To this day, however, they remain part of the antidepressant arsenal.

MAO inhibitors are particularly effective for treating atypical depression, which may be marked by oversleeping, overeating, and anxiety. Examples of MAO inhibitors currently in use include phenelzine sulfate (Nardil) and tranylcypromine sulfate (Parnate).

The next major class of antidepressant drugs, called the tricyclics, was developed in the late 1950s and dominated the antidepressant market for 20 years. Doctors still prescribe them today, although far less frequently. Tricyclics work by desensitizing neuron (nerve) receptors that absorb norepinephrine and serotonin. The result is higher levels of these chemicals in the brain, which causes mood to improve.

Examples of tricyclics include imipramine hydrochloride (Tofranil), amitriptyline hydrochloride (Elavil, Endep), desipramine hydrochloride (Norpramin), doxepin hydrochloride (Sinequan), nortriptyline hydrochloride (Pamelor, Aventyl), and protriptyline hydrochloride (Vivactil).

The newest class of antidepressants are the selective serotonin re-uptake inhibitors (SSRIs).

These work by desensitizing neuron receptors that normally would absorb serotonin—the brain's natural antidepressant. As a result, the brain retains a greater supply of serotonin, which enhances mood and reduces depressive symptoms.

The best known SSRI is Prozac (fluoxetine hydrochloride). Since it went on the market in 1987, Prozac has become the most widely prescribed drug in history. More than 6 million Americans use it regularly, and sales in 1995 amounted to $1.2 billion.

Other SSRIs include Zoloft (sertraline hydrochloride) and Paxil (paroxetine hydrochloride).

Without a doubt, pharmaceutical antidepressants have helped millions of people to overcome the crippling symptoms of depression. Nonetheless, synthetic drugs tend to come with a laundry list of side effects.

Tricyclics, for example, may cause irregular heartbeat, dizziness, fatigue, drowsiness, dry mouth, blurred vision, confusion, hallucinations, weight gain, flu-like symptoms, sweating, rashes, nausea, constipation or diarrhea, difficult urination, sexual dysfunction, and anxiety.

MAO inhibitors may cause orthostatic hypotension (dizziness upon rising from a sitting or reclining position), sedation, dizziness, insomnia, constipation, irregular heartbeat, agitation, fluid retention, sexual dysfunction, weight gain, uncontrollable muscle movement, and muscle cramps. MAO inhibitors may also precipitate a dangerous elevation in blood pressure if combined with foods or medications containing the amino acid tyramine. Foods that are rich in tyramine include aged and cured meat and aged cheese, alcoholic beverages, anchovies, fava beans, liver, pepperoni, pickled foods, and soy sauce.

Among the many drugs that should not be taken in conjunction with MAO inhibitors are amphetamines, antihistamines, decongestants, and other antidepressant medications.

Of the pharmaceutical antidepressants, the SSRIs carry the lowest risk of side effects. Only 17 percent of people who try Prozac stop because of negative experiences, compared to nearly a third of people on tricyclics. Symptoms reported by people who have had adverse reactions to Prozac include nausea (21 percent), headaches (20 percent), anxiety and nervousness (15 percent), insomnia (14 percent), drowsiness (12 percent), diarrhea (12 percent), dry mouth (9 percent), loss of appetite (9 percent), sweating and tremors (8 percent), and rashes (3 percent).

But some doctors question the extent of Prozac's side effects. "I believe that these percentages are far too low and that the true incidence of side effects is much higher," says Hyla Cass, M.D., assistant clinical professor of psychiatry at the UCLA School of Medicine in Los Angeles.

Prozac also has a reputation for causing restlessness in some people who take it. Thus, some physicians must prescribe a second drug to help those people to sleep. Agitation is so pronounced in some cases that Peter Breggin, M.D., co-author of *Talking Back to Prozac*, thinks the drug should be classed as a dangerous, potentially addictive stimulant.

It's also a puzzling fact that many commonly prescribed medications—including remedies for anxiety and emotional distress—may actually cause depression.

Pharmaceutical Pitfalls

Sarah survived the Holocaust, came to the United States, and raised four children with her husband. But as Sarah grew older, painful injuries she had received in concentration camps flared up, so her doctor gave her large doses of painkillers. The drugs alleviated Sarah's physical pain but left her feeling empty and depressed. Sarah found relief only after she stopped taking most of her medications.

"Many physical and psychological problems can be cleared up simply by changing, reducing, or eliminating medicines, if it is appropriate to do so," says Arnold Fox, M.D., the Beverly Hills, California-based physician who treated Sarah. "I'm often horrified at the number of drugs some of my patients have been taking. Far too many doctors find it easier to push pills than to work with patients in setting up lifelong programs of sound mental and physical health."

A variety of medications used to treat other medical problems may cause or worsen depression. Among them are the benzodiazepines, such as alprazolam (Xanax), diazepam (Valium), chlordiazepoxide (Librium), clonazepam (Klonopin), and triazolam (Halcion); phenothiazines, such as prochlorperazine (Compazine) and chlorpromazine (Thorazine); diuretics, digitalis, and several other drugs used to treat cardiovascular disease; indomethacin (Indocin), which is commonly used to treat arthritis pain; oral contraceptives; and some antibiotics. So if you suspect you are suffering from depression, it is important to ask your doctor if any of the medications you take could be causing it.

Moreover, some studies suggest that antidepressant drugs are of little value in treating about 33 percent of depression cases. In one study, antidepressants were only a little more effective than placebos in diminishing symptoms. In another study, patients taking a placebo did just as well as patients on Prozac.

"Antidepressants are only one group of tools we can use to fight depression," Fox says. "They should be used when necessary, but, if possible, reduced or eliminated as nutritional, stress-management, and other techniques begin to take effect."

Using St. John's Wort

For the past 15 years, Fox has been recommending St. John's wort to patients with mild to moderate depression. "I like it," he says, "because its side effects are very mild, especially when compared with the side effects of depression."

Scott Shannon, M.D., a psychiatrist in Fort Collins, Colorado, also reports success in treating depressed patients with St. John's wort. "It elevates mood and raises energy without causing side effects," he says. "Patients tell me they feel brighter, less fatigued, and more able to manage."

St. John's wort has been a popular drug in Europe for years. In Germany, where its use is covered by health insurance as a prescription drug, millions of people take preparations containing St. John's wort.

"St. John's wort isn't something they've just discovered across the Atlantic," says Harold Bloomfield, M.D., an advocate of the herb. "It's been used by European and German physicians in a continuous pattern since ancient times. It comes as a surprise to us here in the United States because we've chosen to sever our roots to herbal medicine."

Among St. John's wort's chemical constituents are tannins, flavonoids, xanthones, terpenes, phloroglucinol derivatives, and carotenoids. Hypericin, a principle component, contains the chemicals that reportedly alleviate depression, although other constituents may play a role as well. But how St. John's wort works remains unclear.

Early research in test tubes indicated that St. John's wort functions much as an MAO inhibitor. Thus, doctors advised patients who consumed the herb to shy away from tyramine-rich foods and medications. Newer studies, however, appear to indicate that this may not be the case. Instead, scientists now say that St. John's wort functions more like an SSRI, blocking re-uptake of serotonin. Still, it might be wise for people who take St. John's wort to at least limit their intake of tyramine-containing substances (see page 17).

In whatever way St. John's wort carries out its biological functions, evidence is sound that the herb is effective in relieving mild to moderate symptoms of depression.

There have been at least 16 randomized, double-blind studies comparing St. John's wort, or *Hypericum*, with a placebo. In 13 of those studies, researchers noted a statistically significant improvement among patients who took *Hypericum*.

In a German study, 15 depressed women took St. John's wort and noted an increase in appetite, greater interest in life, improved feelings of self-worth, and more normal sleep patterns.

Prescription for St. John's Wort

Tea: Steep 1 to 2 teaspoons of the dried herb in a cup of boiling water for 10 to 15 minutes. Drink up to three cups a day. St. John's wort tea first tastes sweet, then later becomes bitter and astringent. Thus, you may want to sweeten your brew with honey.

Tincture: Add ¼ to 1 teaspoon to a glass of hot water up to three times a day. A good quality tincture made from fresh flowering tops will be blood red.

A 1984 clinical trial of St. John's wort involved six depressed women aged 55 to 65. Researchers measured the women's metabolites of noradrenaline and dopamine. After taking *Hypericum* extract, the women showed a marked increase in 3-methoxy-4-hydroxyphenylglucol, which is a chemical marker for antidepressive reactions.

One of the most impressive tests took place in Germany in 1993. Seventy-two patients from 11 doctors' practices were tested on the Hamilton Depression Scale (HAM-D), which measures severity of depression. Then half of the group received St. John's wort; the other half, a placebo (sugar pill). The patients were retested at two and four weeks.

Patients taking St. John's wort demonstrated significant improvement; HAM-D scores fell

---

Capsules: For depression, take 300 milligrams, standardized to at least 0.3 percent hypericin, three times a day.

Caution: Don't give St. John's wort to children younger than 2. For older children and people older than 65, halve the dosage and increase later if necessary. In these two age groups, it is especially important to consult your health-care provider before treating with St. John's wort.

---

from an average of 21.8 to 9.2 after four weeks of treatment, a drop of nearly 60 percent. Inexplicably, the placebo group also noted improvement. But their average HAM-D scores fell only by about 30 percent, from 20.4 to 14.7

The researchers concluded that, "because of its potent and specific efficacy, with few or no side effects, *Hypericum* extract can be recommended as an antidepressant."

How Does St. John's Wort Compare?

There have been at least eight randomized double-blind studies—and scores of less-structured experiments—comparing *Hypericum* with antidepressant drugs such as imipramine, amitryptiline, maprotiline, and desipramine in patients suffering mild to moderate depression. In general, *Hypericum* has produced similar antidepressant effects that appear to grow stronger with length of treatment and have few adverse side effects.

Those findings prompted the *British Medical Journal* to write: "St John's wort is a promising treatment for depression. *Hypericum* extracts were significantly superior to placebos, and similarly effective as standard antidepressants. This herb may offer an advantage in terms of relative safety and tolerability, which might improve patient compliance."

Michael A. Jenike, M.D., editor of the *Journal of Geriatric Psychiatry and Neurology,* agreed in a 1994 report. "The many studies form an impressive body of evidence," Jenike writes. "Treatment with *Hypericum* has been confirmed to have similar effectiveness as synthetic antidepressant drugs. Its mild side effect profile may make it the first treatment of choice for mild to moderate depression."

At the Psychiatric Clinic in Darmstadt, Germany, 135 patients aged 18 to 75 were given either *Hypericum* extract or imipramine three times a day for six weeks. The patients then were tested for depression with the Hamilton Depression Scale and the Clinical Global Impressions Scale (CGI).

The mean HAM-D score fell from 20.2 to 8.8 in the *Hypericum*-treated group and from 19.4 to 10.7 in the imipramine-treated group. The CGI score, which measures therapeutic effectiveness, rose from 1.3 to 3.1 in the *Hypericum* group and from 1.2 to 2.7 in the group of subjects taking imipramine.

Adverse side effects were reported by eight patients on *Hypericum* and 11 patients on imipramine. But the reactions noted by *Hyper-*

icum takers were less severe than those reported by imipramine patients.

Another randomized double-blind study compared *Hypericum* with amitriptyline, given three times a day for six weeks to 80 patients with mild to moderate depression. The HAM-D score fell from 15.82 to 6.34 in the *Hypericum* group and from 15.26 to 6.86 in the amitriptyline group. There were twice as many complaints about adverse effects in the amitriptyline group—58 percent compared to 24 percent among *Hypericum* takers.

Yet another study, performed in 1993, compared the effectiveness of St. John's wort with the tricyclic antidepressant maprotiline. Maprotiline elevates levels of norepinephrine but does not change serotonin levels. This is the opposite of what Prozac does. Maprotiline is also known for working especially quickly. Usually, patients' symptoms begin to disappear just a week or two after beginning treatment with maprotiline, compared with four to eight weeks for St. John's wort.

The study followed the progress of 102 patients at six doctors' practices for four weeks. On average, the patients' initial HAM-D scores were about 21, which indicates moderate depression. Half of the patients received St. John's wort; the other half, maprotiline. Because maprotiline.

works so quickly, patients in that group were the first to notice improvements. But at the end of four weeks, after St. John's wort had time to take effect, improvement in HAM-D scores was identical for both groups: 50 percent.

Potential Problems

St. John's wort is not without its drawbacks. "It can take two to three months to be effective," notes German physician and phytotherapist Rudolph Fritz Weiss, M.D.

Also, says Cass, St. John's wort's influence is much more subtle than pharmaceuticals'. "Most clinicians I've interviewed," she says, "feel that St. John's wort is not quite as potent as [synthetic] drug treatment."

It's true that St. John's wort doesn't work for everyone. Debilitating depression and bipolar disorder (manic-depressive illness) do not respond well to the herb.

"St. John's wort only seems to work on mild to moderate depression," says Fox. "Someone who is severely depressed should be seen by a physician."

And, though most people who take St. John's wort report no adverse reactions, some patients do develop side effects, such as photosensitivity (increased sensitivity of the skin to sunlight), fatigue, gastrointestinal discomfort, anxiety, dizziness, skin rashes and itching, allergy, and heart palpitations. These side effects, however, appear to be mild and rare.

What is unclear, however, is the long-term safety of St. John's wort. No formal studies have evaluated the use of St. John's wort for longer than eight weeks. In Germany, where many people have used the standardized extract during the last 10 years, there have been no reports of fatal reactions to the extract and an extremely low incidence of side effects, which are generally quite mild. That doesn't mean that side effects from long-term use won't show up years down the road, of course.

Nonetheless, a growing number of clinicians conclude that, for most patients, St. John's wort is a safe and effective short-term treatment for mild to moderate depression.

Bear in mind, however, that depression is a serious condition, and left untreated, it can be extremely destructive mentally, physically, and socially. It's important to consult a medical professional if you suspect you have depression, whether or not you are considering taking St. John's wort. A professional can determine if your depression is a result of a physical problem, such as a thyroid hormone imbalance, or a side effect of a medication you take, in which case the depression may be better remedied by treating the underlying disorder or adjusting the medication. A medical professional can also help you determine what type of help is best for your particular situation.

If you have already been diagnosed with depression and are taking a pharmaceutical antidepressant, do not suddenly stop taking it or begin taking St. John's wort along with it. Discuss with your health-care practitioner the possibility of trying St. John's wort; if your practitioner approves, you will likely be weaned off of the pharmaceutical gradually to prevent any major reactions.

Fox says that it's imperative to seek professional help if your depression lingers for more than a couple of weeks or appears to get worse. His reasons go beyond the medication aspects of treatment.

"The cause of the depression is still there and needs to be addressed through counseling," says Fox. "Otherwise, it will resurface throughout your life, regardless of what medicine you are taking."

VALERIAN & MELATONIN FOR INSOMNIA

If you're like most people, you've spent at least one seemingly endless night tossing and turning. Insomnia is one of the most common complaints in our stress-filled society. Although prescription and over-the-counter sleeping pills will help to send you off to dreamland, some of them can have dangerous and even life-threatening side effects. That's why more sleepless consumers are reaching for natural remedies such as valerian and melatonin. The question is: Do they work?

Herbalist David Hoffmann, past president of the American Herbalist Guild, calls valerian "one of the most useful relaxing herbs." Most Europeans would agree. More than 100 drugs based on valerian and its derivatives are marketed in Germany alone. Now valerian preparations are beginning to turn up in medicine cabinets across the United States.

Even more popular with American consumers is a hormone called melatonin. Melatonin has been available in this country for several years. But recent reports touting melatonin as a supplement that can prevent everything from jet lag to old age have sent consumers flocking to pharmacies and health-food stores. Each year, more than 20 million Americans spend millions on melatonin supplements.

How could we resist, when *Newsweek* introduced a recent article on melatonin like this: "It's the hot sleeping pill, natural and cheap. Now scientists say this hormone could reset the body's aging clock, turning back the ravages of time."?

Arnold Fox, M.D., a physician in Beverly Hills, California, who practices conventional and alternative medicine, frequently prescribes melatonin and valerian for his elderly patients.

"Just about every older person has some form of insomnia at one time or another," Fox says. "I really like melatonin because it promotes sleep and is a wonderful antioxidant [a substance that helps the body neutralize free radicals, which are unstable molecules that can damage DNA]. Valerian is also a fascinating remedy that works differently from melatonin but just as effectively."

But the natural supplements aren't just for older people. Roger, in his 40s, is a frequent traveler who sometimes has trouble getting to sleep. He takes melatonin if he has to cross time zones and says the hormone has helped him to ward off the sluggishness and mental confusion associated with severe jet lag.

"I remember once I went to the [former] Soviet Union and had jet lag so bad I didn't sleep for three days," he says. "Then last year, I traveled for more than 24 hours straight to get to Southeast Asia. I took melatonin the first night and woke up the next day feeling as refreshed as if I had been sleeping in my own bed."

When he's troubled by insomnia at home, Roger says he drinks valerian tea. "My wife can't stand the smell," he concedes, "but it's the best natural sleep aid I've ever encountered."

Sleepless in Seattle — and Everywhere Else

Roger's sleep problems are by no means unique. Some experts estimate that more than a million people in the United States have sleep problems at some time — about a third of whom experience chronic insomnia. Twice as many women as men characterize themselves as insomniacs. And, because sleep patterns change as we age, sleep disorders frequently plague the elderly.

Doctors recognize three types of insomnia. People with sleep-onset insomnia have trouble falling to sleep. Those with sleep-maintenance insomnia have trouble staying asleep. And those who have early-awakening insomnia wake long before the rooster crows.

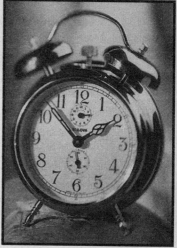

Insomnia is one of the most common complaints in our stress-filled society.

Many factors can contribute to insomnia: anxiety, inappropriate use of medication, conditions such as restless legs syndrome, poor diet, and lack of exercise.

And for every reason you can't fall asleep, it seems, there are a hundred home remedies for correcting the problem: counting sheep, drinking a mug of warm milk, reading a dull book.

Many such remedies can work for cases of mild insomnia. Milk, for example, contains a sleep-inducing amino acid called tryptophan. And counting sheep takes your mind off the anxiety you feel about not being able to sleep.

But occasionally—and, more often than not, it seems, when we have an important appointment or crucial presentation to make at the office the next morning—nothing seems to lull us to sleep. Then we may find ourselves reaching for a pill bottle.

Dangerous Dreams

Each year 4 million to 6 million Americans receive prescriptions for sedative hypnotics. More than half a dozen prescription sleep aids on the market today contain benzodiazepines, which work by reducing the brain's activity, thus helping you to fall asleep.

Melatonin at a Glance

Description: Melatonin is a hormone produced in the body's pineal gland.

Actions: Melatonin affects the body's circadian rhythms, which regulate sleep and waking activities. Melatonin also appears to have strong antioxidant properties.

Uses: Melatonin is used as a natural remedy for jet lag and insomnia.

Possibilities: Some researchers think melatonin may be useful for slowing the aging process and preventing and treating cancer.

"For short-term use, these are very effective sleeping agents," says psychiatry professor Matthew A. Menza, M.D., director of the Consultation Psychiatry Service at Robert Wood Johnson University Hospital in New Brunswick, New Jersey.

However, benzodiazepines have serious drawbacks. For one thing, with fast-acting medications such as zolpidem (Ambien) and triazolam (Halcion), half of their dosage is used up by your body within two to five hours. Thus, you run the risk of waking up in the middle of the night.

Valerian at a Glance

Latin name: *Valeriana officinalis*

Description: This fetid-smelling perennial's family is composed of 200 species. *Valeriana officinalis*, the kind most used in Europe to treat insomnia and anxiety disorders, has a hollow stem and produces small, tubular, pinkish flowers in June.

Habitat: Native to Europe, Asia, and North America, valerian is often found in grasslands, damp meadows, and stream sides, as well as in mountain meadows.

People who tend to wake up frequently might want to try longer-lasting benzodiazepines, such as estazolam (ProSom) or temazepam (Razepam, Restoril). Such medications remain active in your system for about eight hours.

Flurazepam (Dalmane) and quazepam (Doral) remain active for more than 24 hours, making them especially useful for hospitalized patients who need to sleep well and stay relaxed during the day. Daytime drowsiness, however, is undesirable for most people.

If drowsiness were the most serious side effect of benzodiazepines, more people likely would take them. As it is, benzodiazepines and other sleep-inducing medications prescribed by conventional doctors can mask the root cause of a sleep disorder, which could lead to more dangerous health risks and dependencies.

Hypnotic drugs also may cause increased tolerance, dependence, physical addiction, morning hangovers, and withdrawal symptoms if you stop taking them. Another serious side effect is rebound insomnia. After you stop using some drugs, your sleep disorder may actually worsen.

Moreover, if you suddenly stop taking benzodiazepines, you may experience serious withdrawal symptoms. Temazepam's withdrawal effects, for example, may include abdominal and muscle cramps, convulsions, feelings of severe discomfort, inability to fall asleep or stay asleep, sweating, tremors, and vomiting.

Many benzodiazepines can cause depression in susceptible people. Doctors, for example, are warned not to prescribe flurazepam to patients who are severely depressed or have suffered from severe depression.

Drinking alcohol while taking benzodiazepines is extremely dangerous, because alcohol intensifies the effects of the drugs. Thousands of people have died from this deadly combination.

In low doses, antidepressants such as amitriptyline (Amitril, Elavil, Endep) and trazodone (Desyrel) may relieve acute insomnia. But such drugs rarely are a physician's first choice, because they too can cause side effects, the least serious of which include dry mouth and blurred vision.

Over-the-counter sleeping pills have far less serious side effects, but they still may cause problems for some people.

Antihistamines such as hydroxyzine make you drowsy by acting on the central nervous system. They also, of course, will relieve hay fever symptoms, if you have any.

Other over-the-counter sleeping aids include diphenhydramine, dimenhydrinate, and doxylamine.

All of them likely will help you to fall sleep—at first. But after a couple of weeks, most over-the-counter remedies begin to lose their effectiveness. And they don't work at all for people who have serious sleep disorders.

Even more troubling is the warning from Konrad Kail, N.D., past president of the American Association of Naturopathic Physicians. Kail says over-the-counter and prescription sleeping pills appear to alter brain-wave patterns of sleep, thus preventing you from getting the normal cycle of sleep stages needed for optimal health.

Can Valerian Help?

Valerian is a staple medicinal herb used throughout Europe. It's been used for years by Peter Theiss, author of *The Family Herbal* and founder of a large German pharmaceutical herb company.

"Valerian enables you to relax both physically and mentally when you are overworked or experiencing tension and stress," says Theiss. "It does so without making you tired, creating a narcotized sensation, or causing dependency."

Moreover, he says, valerian is much safer than benzodiazepines. "People who easily become irritated or overexcited can use valerian during the day as a gentle sedative as often as they like without detrimental side effects."

Although valerian is just beginning to gain favor with consumers in this country, doctors of yesteryear were quite familiar with this pungent-smelling herb.

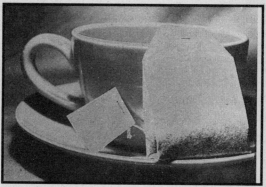

A cup of valerian tea before bed may be the perfect nightcap for people suffering from insomnia.

In 1831, family physician Samuel Thomson wrote: "This powder is the best nervine known. I have made great use of it and have always found it to produce the most beneficial effects in all cases of nervous affection. In fact, it would be difficult to get along in my practice in many cases without this important article."

Today Alan R. Gaby, M.D., former president of the American Holistic Medical Association, recommends valerian for patients with mild to moderate symptoms of insomnia. "For some people only the big guns—the prescription tranquilizers—will offer relief," says Gaby. "But for those with mild insomnia, it's the first thing I try, usually in capsule form."

But Gaby isn't a typical American physician. It's unlikely that many family doctors would recommend valerian to their patients. More doctors, however, may consider valerian after reviewing the clinical evidence that supports the herb's use.

In one double-blind study, 44 percent of insomniacs who took valerian described the quality of their sleep as "perfect," and 99 percent said their sleep had improved significantly. None of the patients reported any side effects.

In another experiment, 128 people with sleep problems were given either 400 milligrams of valerian root extract or a placebo. Those who were taking the herb reported significant improvement in sleep quality without morning grogginess.

Valerian also significantly improves sleep latency, which is how researchers describe the time it takes a person to fall asleep. One study found that valerian halved the time it normally took volunteers to fall asleep.

How exactly does valerian work? "According to the latest information available, we simply don't know," concedes pharmacognosist Varro E. Tyler, Ph.D, professor emeritus at the Purdue University School of Pharmacy in Indiana.

We do know that valerian contains volatile oils, alkaloids, and unstable chemicals known as esters. Esters are lost when valerian root is dried and kept for extended periods. For that reason, the herb's effectiveness may vary considerably, depending on the quality of the brand.

Valerian contains chemicals with strong muscle-relaxant and sedative properties called valepotriates. All parts of the plant contain these chemicals, but they are most concentrated in the roots. Ironically, even valerian preparations without valepotriates have helped some people to fall asleep, raising the possibility that some still unidentified chemical, or a reaction amongst various compounds in the root, may produce a calming effect.

Animal studies conducted in the 1960s demonstrated that valerian acts as a powerful tranquilizer. Subsequent studies with humans replicated those effects. Valerian appears to work by affecting the central nervous system.

Researchers monitored electroencephalograph (a device that measures brain-wave activity) changes in rats that had been given a valerian preparation. They found significant sedative activity, recorded as an increase in brain waves associated with relaxation.

Are They Really Safe?

Valerian: Used in moderation, valerian is safe for most people to take. Extremely large doses of the herb, however, may cause grogginess, vomiting, stupor, and dizziness.

If you use valerian regularly, you could develop a psychological habit, but you won't become physically addicted, as you might with benzodiazepines such as Valium. Withdrawing from valerian use, moreover, causes none of the symptoms associated with stopping benzodiazepines, such as restlessness, insomnia, headache, nausea, and vomiting. In addition, European research indicates that valerian use does not impair your ability to operate machinery, such as an automobile.

Melatonin: The U.S. Food and Drug Administration has reported no adverse reactions from melatonin, but there have been no studies of melatonin's long-term effects.

Thus, it's important to take the supplements as directed, says medical botanist James Duke, Ph.D.,

In another study, a tincture of valerian root was given to 23 hypertensive men. The preparation had a distinct tranquilizing effect, as measured by subsequent brain-wave activity.

Another randomized double-blind study had patients with mild insomnia take either a placebo

former chief of the U.S. Department of Agriculture's Medicinal Plant Laboratory. "Melatonin is a hormone, and in extremely large doses, it could create an imbalance in your body. I would recommend melatonin primarily for jet lag."

Some people have complained that melatonin produces grogginess, extremely vivid dreams, headaches, and mild depression. One study found that melatonin caused mental impairment and drowsiness the day after its use. And some studies with animals suggested a possible carcinogenic effect when it is used during the daytime.

Currently there are no controls over the purity of commercial melatonin preparations. Because there is such a demand for melatonin from consumers, some industry analysts worry that in their rush to supply stores, manufacturers may make production mistakes.

Also, some people may be self-medicating with doses of melatonin that greatly exceed natural levels. In addition, sleep disorders can sometimes indicate a more serious problem, so if you frequently have trouble sleeping, see your doctor before using melatonin.

or an extract of valerian root. Subjective sleep ratings were assessed through a questionnaire, and the patients' movements were recorded throughout the night. The study found that those who took valerian experienced a significant decrease in the amount of time it took them to fall asleep. Higher doses of valerian, interestingly, helped subjects to fall asleep no faster than moderate doses, although clinically it has been observed that higher doses may increase duration of sleep.

Valerian has even been shown in some studies to improve reaction times. And, unlike benzodiazepines, the herb may be taken with alcohol without causing depression or other adverse side effects. Even with prolonged use of valerian, there have been few reports of symptoms such as heartburn, upset stomach, diarrhea, or allergic reactions. Also, unlike sedatives, valerian does not impair one's ability to operate machinery, such as a car.

"Experimental results indicate that valerian root is at least as effective as small doses of barbiturates and benzodiazepines, without the side effects of the latter substances," says Daniel B. Mowrey, Ph.D., author of *Herbs That Heal.*

Herbalists such as Mowrey say valerian is called for primarily when sleep disorders result from anxiety, nervousness, exhaustion, headache, and hysteria.

Melatonin to the Rescue

Melatonin is also proving to be safe and effective, at least for short-term use. Your body comes equipped with a biological clock that regulates sleeping and waking activities. Melatonin, a hormone naturally produced in the body, is believed to help keep the clock ticking by regulating what's known as our circadian rhythm cycle.

Traveling across several time zones disrupts that rhythm, says Richard Dawood, M.D., author of *Travelers' Health: How to Stay Healthy All Over the World*. The result is jet lag, that feeling of exhaustion and disorientation you get when you wake up the next day in a strange hotel room. What may help in those cases is taking melatonin the night before (see "Outsmarting Jet Lag" on page 48).

Our bodies produce melatonin in the bean-size pineal gland nestled deep inside our brains; it is also produced in the retinas of our eyes. Melatonin production is stimulated by darkness and shuts down in the presence of bright light (especially sunlight). Normally, the pineal gland starts increasing its melatonin production around 9 P.M. Hormone levels peak between 2 A.M. and 4 A.M. and then return to their normal daytime levels.

Exactly how melatonin works is unclear. At a worldwide scientific gathering in Switzerland in 1997, Dr. Peretz Lavie reported that electroencephalograms taken during secretion of melatonin are similar to those induced by benzodiazepine drugs such as Klonopin.

But melatonin in no other way resembles benzodiazepines, according to a study that appeared two years earlier in the journal *Psychopharmacology*.

Infants produce a great deal of melatonin. But after we reach puberty, our melatonin levels begin to decrease. As we grow older, the pineal gland calcifies. As a result, "You lose pineal cells, as much as 50 percent," says William Regelson, M.D., a professor of medicine at the Medical College of Virginia at Virginia Commonwealth University in Richmond. "Associated with that loss is a fall in melatonin."

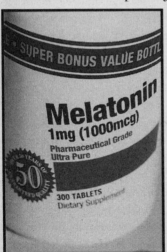

Melatonin is a natural hormone that may aid insomnia sufferers.

By the time we're elderly, melatonin levels are quite low, perhaps accounting for the fact that so many older people suffer from insomnia. Several clinical trials have demonstrated that melatonin-replacement therapy may be beneficial for those people.

Researchers gave a group of elderly insomniacs melatonin and found that the hormone significantly improved sleep maintenance, compared with a placebo (dummy pill).

In another study, 35 elderly insomniacs were given either 2 milligrams of melatonin or a placebo two hours before they went to bed. The groups were tested for two weeks. Those taking melatonin reported the most improvement in sleep patterns.

In a 1995 study in Israel, older people with sleep problems were given melatonin two hours before bedtime for seven days. Then researchers monitored the subjects' sleep and wake patterns. Melatonin, the scientists concluded, was effective for improving sleep maintenance.

A study in the journal *Lancet* suggests that controlled-release melatonin may help older people to stay asleep. Israeli researchers asked 12 people in their 70s and 80s, all of whom weren't producing enough melatonin at night, to take either placebo tablets or tablets that slowly release

2 milligrams of melatonin. After three weeks, the melatonin takers were falling asleep somewhat faster, waking for shorter periods after falling asleep, and spending more time asleep.

Still other studies have confirmed previous reports of melatonin's efficacy:

- A 1994 trial reported in the journal *Neuroreport* found that melatonin helped insomniacs to fall asleep nearly two hours sooner than usual.

- A 1995 study in the *European Journal of Pharmacology* showed that melatonin even improves napping. Young adults were treated with 3 to 6 milligrams of melatonin or a placebo. Those

---

Outsmarting Jet Lag

Don't let jet lag keep you from enjoying your next vacation. To minimize the effects of jet lag, avoid caffeine and alcohol before and during your trip, drink lots of water and juices, and eat light meals.

You could also try melatonin, a supplement available in health-food stores. Melatonin is the hormone your body uses to control its circadian rhythm.

The night before you leave on your trip, take a 3 milligram capsule of melatonin; repeat the dosage the first night you go to sleep in your new destination. If you have more warning of an impending trip, some studies suggest taking 3 milligrams of melatonin in

taking melatonin reported that they were able to get to sleep sooner and stay asleep longer than placebo-taking subjects. The melatonin group members also assessed the quality of their sleep as "deeper" than normal.

• Ten healthy young men were given tablets containing fast-release melatonin, controlled-release melatonin, or a placebo at 11 A.M. In the afternoon, they were asked to take naps. Those taking melatonin reported that the supplement helped them to fall asleep more quickly and to sleep better than usual.

• Researchers gave melatonin to 225 insomniacs and monitored their progress. Within three

---

the afternoon for three days before you leave when flying west to east, then 3 milligrams at night for the first three days you are at your destination. If you are flying east to west, take 3 milligrams each night for three days before you leave, then 3 milligrams in the afternoon for the first three days at your destination. The melatonin will adjust your circadian rhythm and you should wake up feeling fine.

Sunlight also appears to regulate circadian rhythm. If you're traveling east, across up to six time zones, take in bright morning sunlight on the first few days after you arrive. If you're traveling west, expose yourself to sunlight in the late afternoon or early evening. If crossing more than six time zones, avoid bright light until midday.

days, the subjects receiving melatonin reported significantly better quality of sleep and a feeling of "freshness" in the morning.

How Do They Compare?

In trial after trial, valerian seems to work as well as benzodiazepines in helping people to fall asleep. What's more, valerian's sedative effects are not significantly exaggerated by alcohol, as are those from benzodiazepines. And unlike the benzodiazepine Valium, valerian has never been linked to birth defects.

But, for reasons not clearly understood, not all insomniacs respond to valerian. The herb, in fact, seems to mildly stimulate some people.

Prescription for Valerian

Tea: Simmer one teaspoon of powdered root in 1 pint of water for 10 to 15 minutes. Drink one cup about an hour before bedtime. Valerian has an unpleasant taste, so you may want to add honey, lemon, or mint.

Tincture: Take ½ to 1 teaspoon half an hour before bedtime. Repeat if you awaken prematurely.

Capsules: Take as directed, usually one or two capsules half an hour to an hour before bedtime. Repeat if you awaken prematurely.

Like all substances working in the nervous system, valerian has this type of paradoxical effect in a small percentage of people. Such individuals experience this effect beginning with the first dose, and it does not diminish; so, if you do not experience this effect upon taking the first dose of valerian, you can safely assume this effect will not occur at a later time.

In addition, valerian, like other herbs, is not regulated by the federal government. Thus, you can't always be sure about the quality of the valerian product you purchase.

The same holds true for melatonin. Consumers really can't assess the supplement's strength and purity. And, unlike valerian, which has been

Prescription for Melatonin

Capsules: Most people find that 3 milligrams of melatonin taken an hour before bedtime will help them to sleep. If you have trouble staying asleep, you may want to take time-release melatonin capsules. To get the most benefit, the bedroom needs to be totally dark (even the light from a digital clock face can decrease melatonin synthesis). To stop melatonin production in the morning, expose yourself to bright sunlight.

used safely for thousands of years, there have been no studies of the long-term effects of melatonin use. It's also important to note that the beneficial effects of melatonin do not increase with higher dosages. Melatonin should generally be avoided by people suffering from depression. And, there is some evidence from animal studies that melatonin used during the daytime may have a carcinogenic effect.

But based on the clinical evidence so far, both natural remedies certainly seem deserving of further study.

Meanwhile, "I'll continue to use them both," says Roger, the previously sleepless traveler. "It's just not worth the risk to mess around with prescription drugs."

GARLIC FOR HEART DISEASE

A chef whose wit was as sharp as his carving knife once quipped that there are two kinds of people in the world: "People who love garlic, and people who don't know what's good for them." A star ingredient in cuisines from around the world, garlic's pungent taste and aroma send some diners running and cause others to swoon with delight. Whether you love or despise garlic's gastronomic attributes, you may want to add the potent herb to your medicine chest. Scientists are discovering that garlic may hold the key to preventing and treating a number of illnesses, including heart disease.

Don't invite Debbie Hazelton to dinner unless you like to cook with garlic. "I could eat garlic in ice cream," says Hazelton, a psychotherapist and author of *The Courage To See.* "I put it in nearly everything I make—the more the better."

But it's not just the taste that attracts Hazelton to the garlic bulb. An alternative medicine enthusiast, Hazelton values garlic for its medicinal benefits. "From everything I've read," she says, "garlic seems to be a gift from God."

Throughout the ages, nearly every culture on earth has prized garlic. From India and China to Greece and Egypt, ancient healers extolled the healing virtues of garlic. Phoenicians and Vikings carried large stores of garlic to protect them on perilous sea voyages. The Roman scholar Pliny avowed that garlic, first cousin to the ubiquitous onion, was possessed of "very powerful properties," among them the ability to drive away serpents and scorpions. (No studies have substantiated the reactions of poisonous vermin to garlic's overwhelming odor.)

Garlic was also a prime remedy of 19th-century physicians. In 1878, John Gunn, M.D., wrote in the *Home-Book of Health:* "The medicinal uses of garlic are very numerous, it being recommended by some as a valuable expectorant in Consumption and all Affections of the Lungs.... It may be given in the form of a syrup, tincture, or in substances, but the best way to use it when fresh is to express the juice and mix it either with syrup or some other proper vehicle."

In modern times, garlic has been the subject of intensive research in laboratories around the world. And most clinical studies confirm the suspicions of our medical forebears, especially when it comes to treating heart disease. Numerous trials have demonstrated that garlic effectively lowers blood cholesterol and blood pressure. The herb also appears to "thin" blood by inhibiting the excessive clumping of platelets (the blood cells responsible for clotting) and may be useful in preventing heart attacks and strokes.

"Garlic is one of the best heart-healthy herbs around," says Earl Mindell, Ph.D., a registered pharmacologist with a doctorate in nutrition from Pacific Western University and author of *Earl Mindell's Herb Bible*.

Because of its many health attributes, garlic is one of the top-selling herbs in this country, accounting for nearly 6 percent of the $1.27 billion consumers spent on natural health products in 1995.

An Ancient Herb

No one knows how long people have been using garlic. Certainly it ranks among the oldest herbs known to humankind. What records we do have indicate that garlic has been used as a medicine for as long as it has been used to flavor foods.

Garlic's name is believed to derive from the Celtic *gar* for spear or lance, and *lic*, which denotes a leek or type of onion. Garlic's botanical name, *Allium sativum*, comes from the Celtic *all*, which means "smell," and the Latin *sativum*, for "grown" or "cultivated."

But cooks weren't the only ones to use garlic. Medieval herbalist and mystic Hildegarde of Bingen recommended chewing half a garlic clove each day to "invigorate the liver and spleen."

Today researchers such as Gottfried Hertzka, M.D., whose clinic in Konstanz, Germany, has clinically tested more than 500 of Hildegarde's herbal remedies, are looking closely at garlic to determine how useful it may be in treating ailments such as heart disease, the number-one killer in the United States.

Garlic at a Glance

Latin name: *Allium sativum*

Description: A close relative of the onion, garlic produces a compound bulb of up to 15 cloves, which are sheathed in a papery skin that may be tan or pink. Garlic produces small white or pink flowers in spring and summer.

What Is Heart Disease?

In our fast-paced, industrialized world, where stress is as common as the fatty fast foods so many of us consume, two of every five Americans die of heart attacks or degenerative heart and blood vessel diseases.

Among the greatest risk factors for developing cardiovascular disease are high blood pressure, which can be aggravated by obesity, and high blood cholesterol, which often results from consuming too much fat and can lead to the formation of deadly blood clots.

It is those conditions—and many more—that garlic seems capable of preventing and treating.

High blood pressure, or hypertension, is the most common cardiovascular disease in the in-

Habitat: Although it has been used since recorded time, nobody really knows where garlic originated. Some botanists think it may be indigenous to southern Siberia. Today garlic is grown around the world.

dustrialized world. In the United States alone, more than 40 million people have been diagnosed with the condition. You may have high blood pressure and not even know it. The illness rarely causes symptoms. Nonetheless, this so-called silent killer is the leading cause of stroke and a major cause of heart attacks.

Blood pressure refers to the force of blood as it pushes against artery walls. As excessive air pressure can damage a tire, high blood pressure can be harmful to arteries and organs. When blood pressure is consistently high—140/90 or more—the heart is forced to work beyond its capacity. Eventually this vital muscle runs the risk of stretching and losing elasticity, decreasing its ability to pump blood at all.

If your blood pressure is mildly or moderately high, your doctor may ask you to lose excess weight, which will take some of the "load" off your heart. Physicians also recommend cutting back on sodium, which can cause some people to retain water and increase blood pressure. And they suggest that people with hypertension eat lots of fruits and vegetables, which recent studies have shown can help to lower blood pressure.

If lifestyle changes alone don't do the job, your doctor may prescribe any of a number of medications to bring down your blood pressure to an acceptable level. In most cases, the medicines accomplish their tasks. But just as often, blood pressure drugs cause as many problems as they solve.

Diuretics, for example, cause the body to shed excess water, which reduces blood volume and causes a drop in blood pressure. But because they tamper with the kidney's natural processes, diuretics strain the

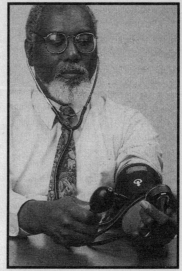

Regular blood pressure checks are vital in order to detect this silent killer.

kidneys, which can lead to serious problems. Diuretics may also worsen diabetes, cause impotence, and significantly increase cholesterol levels. Some diuretics also cause the body to lose potassium, which is necessary to regulate the heart's intricate electrical system.

Beta-adrenergic blockers, another class of drugs, compensate for the effects of high blood pressure by making the heart beat more slowly and with less force. The drugs, however, also may cause decreased sexual ability, depression, difficulty breathing, dizziness, fatigue, insomnia, itching, nightmares, stomach upset, and even congestive heart disease.

Other drugs used to treat high blood pressure include calcium channel blockers, angiotensin-converting enzyme (ACE) inhibitors, and alpha-adrenergic blockers—all of which lower blood pressure by relaxing and dilating arteries. But these, too, can cause problematic side effects. Calcium channel blockers, for example, can cause constipation, dizziness, fatigue, fluid retention, flushing, headache, low blood pressure, nausea, rash, shortness of breath, and slow heartbeat. ACE inhibitors can cause abdominal pain, cough, dizziness, dry mouth, fatigue, headache, irregular heartbeat, itching, loss of taste, low blood pressure, nausea, muscle cramps, rash, and vomiting. And alpha-adrenergic blockers can cause difficult breathing, dizziness, drowsiness, fatigue, headache, heart palpitations, low blood pressure, nasal stuffiness, nausea, wrist and ankle swelling, and weakness.

"Good" and "Bad" Cholesterol

Like high blood pressure, high blood cholesterol produces no noticeable symptoms. You won't know whether your cholesterol is too high unless you have your doctor check it.

If it is too high, you're not alone. Nearly half of all Americans—40 percent—have cholesterol levels that physicians consider to be unhealthy.

Cholesterol is a naturally occurring fatlike substance produced by the human liver and also found in meat, egg yolks, and dairy products. The waxy substance is vital for such physiological functions as building new cells, insulating nerves, and producing hormones.

Cholesterol binds with protein molecules to form various types of substances known as lipoproteins. High-density lipoprotein (HDL) cholesterol is a tiny, dense particle that transports excess cholesterol to the liver, where it is altered and expelled from the body in bile. HDLs are considered beneficial because they help rid the body of excess cholesterol.

Low-density lipoprotein (LDL) cholesterol is a larger particle that tends to remain in the body. When LDL is oxidized (see page 67), it becomes the so-called "bad" cholesterol that clogs arteries, causing atherosclerosis, which can lead to heart attacks.

Whether your cholesterol is high or low—a total blood cholesterol level below 200 is considered safe—depends largely on your genetic makeup, diet, and exercise level. If your cholesterol reading is above acceptable levels, your doctor will likely test your blood to determine if you have a higher than advisable level of LDL cholesterol.

If testing reveals that you have a higher than recommended level of LDL cholesterol, you will most likely be advised to make dietary changes to help lower your blood cholesterol level. Such changes will include not only cutting back on cholesterol-laden foods but lowering the amount of fat—especially saturated fat—in your diet, since a high-fat diet tends to increase LDL cholesterol in your blood. You'll be advised, among other steps, to substitute skim-milk products for whole-milk products; limit fatty meats and trim all visible fat from the meats you do eat; use less oil in cooking and baking; and restrict heavily processed foods and foods containing hydrogenated or partially hydrogenated vegetable oils in your diet. In place of fattier foods, you'll be asked to follow a diet based largely on fresh fruits and vegetables and whole grains, which contain fiber and can help to clean cholesterol from your system. (Your doctor or a registered dietitian can help you plan appropriate changes in your diet.)

Your doctor will also likely recommend that you get regular physical activity, which can help increase HDL cholesterol and help you lose excess weight; being overweight can contribute to problems with blood cholesterol and blood pressure.

If diet and lifestyle changes fail to reduce your LDL cholesterol levels, your doctor may prescribe a drug, such as lovastatin (Mevacor), simvastatin (Zocor), or pravastatin (Pravachol), that blocks an enzyme that the liver uses to manufacture cholesterol.

Other cholesterol-reducing drugs work by attaching themselves to the bile acids in the intestines. Bile encourages the absorption of fat from foods, which in turn increases blood cholesterol. The drugs are indigestible and pass out of the body, taking the bile acids with them.

For many people, cholesterol-reducing drugs have proved to be highly effective. But for some people, they can cause serious side effects. Lovastatin, simvastatin, and pravastatin, for example, have caused liver inflammation in a small number of people.

And in one clinical test, 68 percent of people who took the bile-acid binding drug cholestyramine (Questran) suffered moderate to severe reactions, which included constipation, gas, heartburn, and bloating. Such drugs may also increase the risks of developing gallstones and cancer in some people.

Put Your Blood on a Diet

Lowering unhealthy cholesterol is important for preventing formation of blood clots in the arteries that supply the heart. Such blood clots constitute the leading cause of heart attacks.

Many medications are useful for "thinning" the blood and preventing clots from forming. Aspirin, or acetylsalicylic acid, is commonly prescribed by doctors to do just that.

Although aspirin was discovered in the 19th century, we still don't know exactly how it works. Researchers surmise that aspirin interferes with the production of chemicals called prostaglandins, which regulate numerous functions, including body temperature, pain perception, and blood clotting.

Although aspirin causes at least some microscopic bleeding in the gastrointestinal tract of those who take it regularly, it is safely tolerated by most people. But this common over-the-counter remedy may cause serious and even fatal bleeding in some people. Problems usually result when people take too much aspirin. You need very little aspirin to benefit from the drug's anticlotting properties. Experts recommend one adult aspirin (325 milligrams) taken every other day or one baby aspirin (81 milligrams) taken daily, although some studies suggest that even smaller amounts may be protective.

In trial after trial, garlic has produced no major side effects. But can garlic replace or augment conventional medicines used to prevent and treat some forms of heart disease?

What Garlic Does

Michael Castleman, author of *The Healing Herbs,* minces no words in his praise of garlic's benefits to the cardiovascular system. "No standard medications match garlic when it comes to acting on so many cardiovascular risk factors at the same time," he says.

Castleman bases his assessment on scientific research. Garlic is one of the most widely studied herbs in medical history. In the last 20 years, more than 1,000 scientific papers have noted garlic's powerful effects on the cardiovascular system.

Among the garlic researchers is Eric Block, a professor of chemistry at the State University of New York at Albany. Block reported in 1985 that garlic:

- Lowers total and low-density-lipoprotein cholesterol in the blood.

- Raises high-density-lipoprotein cholesterol.

- Reduces the tendency of blood to clot.

- Offers antioxidant protection to cell membranes.

How does garlic achieve so many healthful effects? Perhaps part of the explanation lies in the fact that garlic contains antioxidants, such as vitamins A and C and the mineral selenium.

To appreciate the value antioxidants have for health, you need to first understand the dangers of oxygen. It is a real mystery of nature that an element as vital to life as oxygen is also one of its most toxic. Actually, the oxygen itself is not the problem; rather, it is a form of oxygen that has been chemically modified into a highly unstable substance called a free radical. A free radical is unstable because one of its parts—called an electron—is missing and must be replaced. So it seeks out other compounds in the body and steals an electron from one of them to restore its stability. If the compound giving up its electron is an LDL molecule, the result is the formation of the fatty streaks in the walls of the blood vessels that are the hallmark of atherosclerosis.

Free radicals form in a number of ways, and many of the forces that cause them cannot be stopped. They are formed in the normal course of metabolism, for example. In fact, it is impossible to avoid them, since our metabolism is based on oxygen. The body has a means for handling a normal burden of free radicals. Antioxidants are the weapons the body uses for protection against damage from free radicals. It is only when the production of free radicals overwhelms the body's protective system of antioxidants that disease-producing damage results.

The heart and the blood vessels, like the lungs, are especially vulnerable to the toxic effects of oxygen because their exposure to this element is so great. The blood is the route of transport for oxygen throughout the body. The blood is also the route of transport for many of the substances that can act on oxygen to produce free radicals. Cholesterol is also carried through the blood packaged in LDL particles. And it is the LDL that is responsible for depositing cholesterol in the walls of the arteries. These deposits form fatty build-ups that eventually narrow the arteries, possibly leading to a heart attack. Scientists now know that before LDL cholesterol can have this effect, it first has to be modified by a free radical to form an oxidized LDL. In other words, the free radical substances produced in the blood from oxygen by any one of a number of causes, like chemicals from cigarette smoke, can set off a chain of events generating oxidized LDL cholesterol and ultimately lead to heart disease.

Antioxidants protect LDL cholesterol against damage by free radicals either by preventing them from forming or by destroying them once they have formed. Antioxidants also protect against heart disease by reducing the tendency for blood clots to form. A blood clot may eventually plug an artery narrowed by fatty plaques, thereby cutting off the supply of oxygen to a portion of the heart and bringing on a heart attack.

Another potential key player in garlic's healing nature is a sulfur-containing compound called allicin, which gives garlic its odor. When fresh garlic is crushed, two substances are released — the compound alliin and the enzyme allinase. These two react to form allicin. Allicin boosts levels of two blood enzymes with antioxidant properties: catalase and glutathione peroxidase.

In recent years, scientists have discovered other sulfur-containing compounds in garlic, including S-allyl cysteine, ajoene, vinyldithiins, and (gamma)-glutamyl S-allyl cysteine. These chemicals also appear to be protective, although they are less well understood.

How Garlic Lowers Blood Pressure

"Garlic is wonderful for bringing down high blood pressure," says John Heinerman, Ph.D., a medical anthropologist and expert on healing foods. "It has to be one of the most useful herbs for doing so in the entire plant kingdom. I know of nothing else that works so rapidly or so well for this common problem."

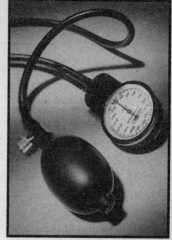
Garlic can help reduce blood pressure.

Scores of studies validate Heinerman's assessment. Experiments at Sandoz Pharmaceuticals in Switzerland dating back to the 1920s, for example, confirm garlic's ability to reduce blood pressure in animals and humans.

In 1929, German researchers noted consistent reductions in blood pressure in 80 hypertensive patients who were treated with garlic. The study was replicated in 1931. The researchers also found that garlic tincture caused a marked drop in blood pressure.

In 1948, Swiss researchers found that garlic reduced blood pressure by a significant amount in more than 40 percent of cases. The scientists used every precaution in order to ensure that the drop in blood pressure was due solely to the administration of garlic. Regardless of how old the patients were or how high their blood pressure readings were, garlic worked across the board.

Garlic appears to lower blood pressure by dilating, or expanding, the blood vessels. Think of it like this: If you step on a garden hose, you increase the pressure of water flowing through the hose. Take your foot off of the hose—effectively dilating it—and the water pressure returns to normal. But how does garlic work to expand blood vessels?

Garlic contains chemicals called adenosine deaminase and cyclic AMP phosphodiesterase. Recently, researchers discovered that those

Is Garlic Really Safe?

Most people can take all the garlic they want. But because garlic "thins" the blood, people on anticlotting medications, such as warfarin (Coumadin) or aspirin, should be careful about how much garlic they consume (check with your doctor). As with anything, garlic may cause an allergy or rash in sensitive people. And some people complain that garlic upsets their stomachs.

chemicals are capable of inhibiting certain enzymes. The presence of such enzyme inhibitors in garlic may help to explain several of garlic's clinical effects, including its ability to dilate blood vessels.

Garlic and Cholesterol

Studies also suggest that garlic effectively gets rid of "bad" cholesterol, while it increases levels of "good" cholesterol. A number of trials in India credit garlic with significantly reducing blood cholesterol levels and "cleaning up" clogged arteries.

In a 1973 experiment published in the British medical journal *Lancet*, researchers asked volunteers to eat a meal containing four ounces of butter, which is known to raise blood cholesterol

If you want to try garlic as an adjunct to current treatment for cardiovascular disease, be sure to discuss this with your doctor. And do not stop taking any prescribed medication for cardiovascular disease (even low-dose aspirin) unless your physician advises you to do so.

levels. Half of the group also ate nine cloves of garlic. Three hours later, the average cholesterol level among people who did not eat garlic jumped 7 percent. But the cholesterol levels of garlic eaters dropped 76 percent. The researchers concluded that, "garlic has a very significant protective action [against high blood cholesterol]."

Garlic and Blood Clots

By inhibiting harmful LDL cholesterol, garlic may help you to prevent blood clots. Another way it may inhibit clots is to thin the blood. Some researchers think that garlic is at least as potent as aspirin but with none of aspirin's side effects.

Prescription for Garlic

Try adding a clove or more of fresh—preferably raw—garlic to your daily menu.

Or, if you want to try a commercial garlic preparation, try taking 500 to 1,500 milligrams of a garlic extract standardized to 1 milligram allicin each day. And don't fall for manufacturers' claims of odor-free garlic pills. If you and your doctor decide you need high-allicin garlic, it's going to have an odor. If garlic breath is a concern, try taking supplements with

How are clots formed? A protein called fibrin is essential to the clotting of blood. Without it, the blood will not coagulate (thicken to form a clot). Garlic is able to split or divide this protein so that harmful blood clots don't form. Allicin and adenosine appear to be the most potent antiplatelet constituents of garlic.

What Kind of Garlic Should You Take?

It's unclear exactly how much garlic you need to consume—and in what form—to help protect your heart and blood vessels. Some experts suggest you'd need to eat at least five cloves a day, while others think that a clove a day provides a protective effect. If you enjoy the taste of garlic,

---

an enteric coating, which causes odor-producing allicin and allinase to break down in the small intestine instead of the stomach. Eating parsley or other greens with a high chlorophyll content after you've consumed garlic also will help lessen the smell.

Remember, too, that whether you take garlic or prescription medications, it's essential that you adopt healthy lifestyle habits, such as avoiding cigarette smoke, getting plenty of physical activity, and eating a low-fat, high-fiber diet. No single food or pharmaceutical can make up for poor health habits.

a clove a day would probably be a fairly easy prescription to fill. However, even garlic lovers—and those near them—would likely balk at having to consume five or more cloves on a daily basis.

Some people, therefore, have turned to garlic supplements. In general, garlic products fall within two categories: aged garlic extract and high-allicin garlic supplements. Proponents of the latter say it's the allicin that delivers garlic's multiple health benefits. If you buy this kind of garlic, don't be fooled by claims that it's odor free. Allicin is what gives garlic its odor, so an odor-free supplement logically would contain no allicin.

Now what about aged garlic extract? Studies show that this type of garlic lacks the herb's bacteria- and virus-killing properties. But other studies indicate that compounds formed during the aging process—S-allyl-cysteine and S-allyl-mercapto-cysteine, in particular—are strong immune-system enhancers and can help to prevent some illnesses.

A 1997 study that appeared in *Phytotherapy Research* showed that aged garlic boosts cellular superoxide dismutase (SOD) levels and enhances glutathione. Thus, they conclude that aged garlic extract may help the body to stave off aging-related diseases, including atherosclerosis, by increasing the body's ability to neutralize free radicals.

However, two recent studies found no beneficial effect on blood cholesterol levels from taking garlic supplements. One study tested daily supplements of dried, powdered garlic equal to about a clove and a half of fresh garlic; the other study tested daily supplements of garlic oil equal to about a clove and a half's worth of garlic. Both studies lasted four months.

Until further research can confirm the benefits of commercial garlic supplements, you may want to opt for simply adding more fresh garlic to your meals, such as in salads and other dishes. That way, you are more likely to garner all of the potential benefits of garlic—no matter which components end up being most effective for disease prevention.

Consider Hazelton's assessment. "Garlic just plain tastes good," she says. "If everyone ate it, the world would be a better place."

ECHINACEA FOR COLDS & FLU

*Every school child knows that the contributions
made by American Indians to the first
Thanksgiving—including corn and
beans—helped to save the lives of early
colonists. Today, we can add echinacea
to that list of Native gifts. The Plains
Indians used echinacea to treat just
about everything. Now, research has
confirmed that echinacea contains
chemicals that spur the body to heal itself.
That's important when you consider
that pharmaceuticals are basically useless in
treating that most common infection—the cold.*

The Indians considered echinacea to be nothing
less than a panacea. The Sioux Indians applied
a freshly scraped echinacea root as a poultice to
treat the bites of rabid animals. The Cheyenne
used echinacea to heal mouth ulcers. Choctaws
took echinacea when they came down with a
bad cough. And Delaware Indians used echinacea to treat venereal diseases.

"Echinacea was used more than any other plant by Indians in the Plains states," says anthropologist Melvin Gilmore.

Other tribes employed the plant to treat rheumatism, infections, bee stings, indigestion, tumors, gangrene, eczema, hemorrhoids, wounds, insect bites, painful teeth and gums, smallpox, measles, mumps, arthritis, colds, and snakebites.

Few modern Americans have use for snakebite remedies. But more and more of us are turning to echinacea as a natural remedy for colds and flu. Once confined to health-food stores and mail-order catalogs, echinacea remedies increasingly are showing up on the shelves of conventional pharmacies.

Nature's Way, for example, makes a popular product called EchinaGuard, and Enzymatic turns out EchinaFresh, both of which rely on echinacea as a main ingredient. Other companies marketing popular echinacea remedies include HerbPharm, Gaia, Eclectic Institute, and McZand.

Echinacea's current popularity would probably come as no surprise to your great-grandmother. In her day, nearly every medicine cabinet contained echinacea in one form or another. But the discovery of antibiotics in the 1930s overshadowed the regard that physicians once held for the herb, and echinacea rapidly lost favor with consumers.

Now, as scientists tell us that antibiotics may be losing their effectiveness in fighting germs, researchers are taking another look at echinacea. In particular, they're interested in echinacea's ability to fight off infections.

What Is an Infection?

In the course of the average day, you're exposed to legions of germs, including bacteria and viruses. You can pick up pathogens (agents that cause disease) by touching germ-infested objects, breathing contaminated air, or eating food or drinking beverages that have been exposed to germs. Pathogens also may invade our bodies through sexual contact or through insect and animal bites.

Echinacea at a Glance

Latin names: *Echinacea angustifolia, Echinacea purpurea*

Description: Echinacea is a lovely perennial. Its stout, sturdy stems are covered with bristles, and its roots are

Your body comes equipped with natural barriers to germs. Your skin, for example, is there to stop germs from invading your organs. If a pathogen manages to get past your skin and inside your body, it will attempt to survive by attacking healthy cells and reproducing. Most germs succumb to your body's array of disease-fighting white blood cells. Others are expelled in mucus, sweat, and other waste products. Germs that do survive prey on healthy cells and tissues. The result is an infection, and symptoms may include fever, chills, sweating, headache, muscle pain, nasal congestion, and fatigue.

Now it's up to your immune system to come to the rescue. The immune system is your body's defense department. When the immune system is alerted to the presence of pathogenic invaders, it calls out a veritable army of infection fighters. Proteins called antibodies team up with special white blood cells to neutralize and destroy pathogens. When white blood cells called

long and black on the outside. Its cone-shaped flower heads, which appear mid- to late summer, are composed of numerous tiny purple florets surrounded by deep pink petals.

Habitat: Native to the American prairies from southern Canada to Texas, echinacea is often found on flat lands, in open woods, in fields, and on roadsides.

neutrophils gather at infection sites, you experience the achiness and inflammation that accompany infections.

The immune system is also able to remember whether it's ever encountered a particular pathogen. That way, it automatically knows how to suppress repeat invaders. This cellular memory, sometimes aided by vaccines, gives the body immunity against countless disease-causing agents.

Immune system responses stop or weaken most, but not all, infections. Sometimes immune cells fail to recognize and attack pathogens, especially if they're new to the body. At other times, the body's counterattack simply isn't enough to ward off the invaders.

People whose immune systems are weakened by fatigue, poor nutrition, certain medical treatments (such as radiation therapy), or illnesses (such as Acquired Immune Deficiency Syndrome) are more susceptible to infection than are people in generally good health.

Ah-Choo!

Nancy, a church administrator and mother of two, never used to get colds until the children came along. "Now," she says, "they bring home every cold bug that makes its way into their school."

At first, Nancy turned to over-the-counter remedies or simply suffered as she went about her work. Then a friend told her about echinacea, and she's been using it ever since.

"I take it the minute one of my kids sneezes," she says, "and almost always I'm able to ward off most of the symptoms I'd otherwise have for a week."

The common cold is the most frequent infection in all age groups in the United States. A cold results when a virus attaches itself to the lining of your nasal passages or throat.

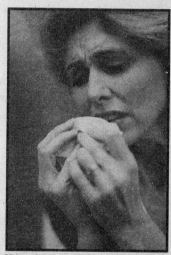

Using tissues can help stop the spread of a cold virus.

The cold virus can be acquired through airborne particles when an infected person sneezes or coughs near you. More often, though, the virus is picked up when you touch an object contaminated with secretions from an infected person's mucous membranes and then touch your own nose or mouth. For example, you can get the cold virus on your hand by shaking hands with a cold sufferer who has recently sneezed into his hand or by touching a doorknob that a cold sufferer has touched after wiping her nose. Then, when you touch your own nose or mouth, the virus gains entry to your body. (That's why using disposable tissues and washing your hands frequently can help prevent the spread of colds.)

Your immune system responds to this viral invasion by sending out its white-blood-cell soldiers. Your body's immune responses actually cause the symptoms of the cold, which, depending on its severity, can include head and chest congestion, runny nose, difficulty breathing, sore throat, sneezing, coughs, chills, and fatigue.

Once you have caught a cold caused by a particular virus, your white blood cells recognize that invader and will prevent future colds by that same marauder. Unfortunately, there are more than 200 different viruses that cause colds, so just because you gain protection from one, doesn't mean the others won't get you.

Influenza causes many of the same symptoms as the common cold, only they're usually much more severe. And, like the cold virus, the flu virus can be contracted by inhaling contaminated droplets in the air or by handling items touched by someone who's been infected. Symptoms generally develop from one to four days after your initial contact with the virus.

There are three general categories of flu-causing viruses. Researchers call them types A, B, and C. All three types of virus can mutate, or change form (although B and C are somewhat more stable than A), so you can never develop a permanent immunity to influenza. Many of the influenza viruses that infect us seem to originate in parts of Asia, where close contact between people and livestock creates an environment conducive to viral growth.

Influenza makes most of us miserable at one time or another. But for people who are very old, young, or sick, flu can be deadly. Today it's almost impossible to imagine that in 1918 an influenza epidemic that started in a training camp in Kansas spread around the world and killed more than 20 million people. In the United States alone, more than 500,000 people died so quickly that health authorities had a difficult time gathering up the bodies.

What Doctors Tell You

About all that doctors can do for you when you come down with a cold or flu is advise you to rest, eat nourishing foods, and drink plenty of liquids to flush the toxins from your body. As a result, many people turn to over-the-counter medications for relief.

Pain relievers, such as aspirin or acetaminophen, can help ease headaches and body aches and bring down an uncomfortable fever. Children, however, should never be given aspirin. Doing so may trigger Reye syndrome, a neurological disease that can cause coma, brain damage, and death in children under age 18.

Antihistamines, such as chlorpheniramine and diphenhydramine, may stop a runny nose and suppress coughing. These drugs, however, can cause drowsiness, dry mouth, and blurred vision.

Decongestants, such as pseudoephedrine and phenylephrine, can relieve a stuffed-up nose. However, they can cause tremors and heart palpitations and should be avoided by people with high blood pressure or other cardiovascular problems. And when taken in the form of nosedrops or sprays, decongestants can actually cause rebound congestion that is more severe than the original symptom.

But, aside from the potential side effects of over-the-counter cold and flu preparations, there is a greater concern with using these products. As stated previously, the symptoms of a cold or flu are actually your body's response to the invader; they signal your body's attempts to rid itself of the enemy. And since over-the-counter preparations tend to inhibit these symptoms, many experts feel that they can actually prolong your suffering by dampening your body's own ability to heal itself.

As far as prescription medications are concerned, there's not much help available for these viral infections. Antibiotics, such

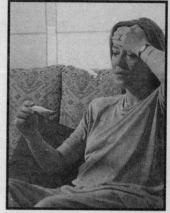

A fever may help your body rid itself of the flu virus.

as penicillin and its derivatives, work extremely well to eradicate certain bacterial infections, but they do nothing to kill viruses. (Indeed, overuse or misuse of antibiotics can suppress the body's natural immune reactions.)

Antiviral medications, such as amantadine and rimantadine, may relieve some symptoms of a viral infection. But up to 30 percent of people are infected by influenza viruses that are resistant to the drug. These drugs also cause side effects that can be more uncomfortable or dangerous to an otherwise healthy flu sufferer than the flu itself; such side effects include confusion, difficulty concentrating, dizziness, headache, irritability, loss of appetite, nausea, nervousness, blotchy spots on the skin, and trouble sleeping.

In terms of medicinal prevention of viral infections, you can get a flu shot. Each year, scientists take an educated guess at which flu strain will be most prevalent and create a vaccine for that specific virus. However, the viruses that cause flu are continuously changing and mutating, so if you come in contact with a virus other than the one targeted by the vaccine, you're likely to get sick.

Echinacea to the Rescue

When it comes to fighting nonviral infections, echinacea is no substitute for punch-packing pharmaceutical antibiotics. But research does support echinacea's effectiveness for some viral infections, such as the cold and flu, because it significantly boosts your body's immune system and helps you to heal faster than you otherwise might.

"In one study, echinacea was shown to prevent and shorten the length of some illnesses," according to medical botanist and herb expert James Duke, Ph.D, former chief of the U.S.

Department of Agriculture's Medicinal Plant Laboratory.

Compared with some other herbal treatments, we know quite a bit about echinacea. In the last 30 years, more than 500 scientific studies have been conducted to determine the herb's safety and efficacy.

The most consistently proven effect of echinacea is in stimulating a process called phagocytosis, which encourages white blood cells to attack invading organisms. Among other scientifically proven actions, echinacea:

- Increases the number and activity of immune system cells, including anti-tumor cells.

- Stimulates new tissue growth to aid in wound healing.

- Reduces inflammation in arthritis and inflammatory skin conditions.

- Induces mild antibiotic action against bacteria, viruses, fungi, and other germs.

- Inhibits the enzyme hyaluronidase, to help prevent bacterial access to healthy cells.

- Slows the spread of infection to surrounding tissues and helps to flush toxins from infected areas.

"The herb normalizes the number of white blood cells in the blood and helps them surround and destroy bacteria and viruses," says Daniel B. Mowrey, Ph.D., director of the American Phytotherapy Research Laboratory in Salt Lake City, Utah, and author of *The Scientific Validation of Herbal Medicine*.

In Germany, extensive research over the past few decades has uncovered a host of echinacea's infection-fighting properties, including the ability to power up the immune system, treat colds and flu, and prevent infection.

Further clinical trials have confirmed those findings and illuminated others.

A 1989 study, for example, found that an extract of echinacea increased immune function by as much as 120 percent over five days. And in 1985, human white blood cells stimulated by an echinacea extract were found to have increased their ability to overwhelm infectious yeast cells by 20 to 40 percent.

Is Echinacea Really Safe?

Echinacea is generally considered safe, although an allergic reaction is always a possibility in some people, says Varro E. Tyler, Ph.D., herb expert and professor emeritus at Purdue University School of Pharmacy in

How Echinacea Works

Echinacea appears to boost the body's immune response. Unlike a vaccine, which is active only against specific invaders, echinacea stimulates overall activity of cells responsible for fighting any infection that exists in your body.

Unlike antibiotics, which simply kill bacteria, echinacea stimulates the body, at a cellular level, to fight off bacteria, viruses, and other pathogens. In other words, echinacea tells your body to heal itself.

Early on, researchers determined that echinacea has a profound effect on the number and kind of blood cells in the bloodstream. Echinacea promotes production of white blood cells when the percentage is too low and helps them get to where they can fight the infection more effectively.

West Lafayette, Indiana. Stop using echinacea if you experience any adverse effects. Some German herbalists say echinacea should not be used in progressive systemic and auto-immune disorders, such as tuberculosis, and connective tissue disorders, such as lupus. Evidence of its efficacy in treating opportunistic infections in AIDS patients, they say, is inconclusive.

We don't know all of the components of echinacea or whether its actions are the result of one or a combination of chemicals. We do know that echinacea roots contain caffeic acid glycoside, which reacts with other substances in the body's cells to promote healing.

Some of echinacea's chemical constituents also appear to be involved in regrowth of connective tissue that has been destroyed during infection, an action that greatly stimulates the healing process.

When germs get into your bloodstream, they stimulate an enzyme called hyaluronidase to break down the connective tissue surrounding cells. Once these connective tissues have been compromised, germs can easily latch onto the cells and begin the progressive cellular destruction known as infection. But studies in Eastern Europe in the 1960s found that echinacea neutralizes hyaluronidase, so the germs can't get a cellular foothold.

Echinacea also helps your body to produce natural infection-fighting chemicals. Your spleen, liver, and lymph nodes contain large white blood cells called macrophages, which filter lymphatic fluid and blood and engulf and destroy bacteria, cellular debris, and other foreign particles in a process called phagocytosis. Before a virus-infected cell dies, it releases a small amount of interferon, which boosts the ability of surrounding cells to resist infection. Echinacea stimulates macrophages to produce interferon and other immune-enhancing compounds, including interleukins, and tumor necrosis factor, which then fight off infections that cause colds, flu, respiratory and urinary tract illness, and other conditions.

Researchers discovered this after bathing cells in echinacea extract and then exposing them to two potent viruses: those that cause influenza and herpes. Unlike the untreated cells, only a small proportion of echinacea-treated cells became infected.

A study in Germany in 1978 found that in the presence of echinacea, viruses and bacteria had a greatly diminished capacity for causing infections. That means the herb either prevents the virus from reproducing or actively competes with the virus for receptor sites on cells to which the pathogen is naturally attracted, thus preventing microbial invaders from gaining entrance to the cells.

Treating Colds

Despite the miraculous advances of modern medicine in recent years, doctors still are powerless to prevent or cure the common cold. But several studies indicate that echinacea may help us to ward off this frequent illness.

A recent double-blind study in Germany looked at echinacea as a preventive treatment against colds and other viral infections. Volunteers were given 4 milliliters of juice squeezed daily from echinacea leaves and flowers.

The results were impressive. Of volunteers participating in the study, 32.5 percent of those taking echinacea remained healthy after exposure to cold viruses, compared to 25.9 percent in a placebo (inactive substance) group.

Prescription for Echinacea

Echinacea root is the part that has historically been used in European and American herbalism. Today, nearly all parts of the plant are used, including the root, leaves, flowers, and seeds. Echinacea is available commercially in a number of forms, including dried root or herb, liquid extract, powder, capsules and tablets, and creams and gels. Echinacea preparations are approved drugs in European countries. The officially recommended usage levels and those used in research studies are:

Tea: Simmer 1 to 2 teaspoons of dried echinacea in 1 cup boiling water for 10 to 15 minutes. Drink up to 3 cups a day.

Those taking echinacea also stayed healthier longer: 40 days, compared to 25 days for people who took placebos. And when infections did occur among the echinacea group members, illnesses were less severe and tended to clear up much more quickly than for placebo takers.

Most herbalists advise taking echinacea the minute you feel a cold coming on, so your body can ward it off before symptoms get a foothold. There's a myth that echinacea loses its effectiveness when used continually. There's no evidence to support this. Indeed, clinical evidence supports its effectiveness in long-term use.

Tincture: Follow manufacturers' directions, usually 1 to 5 droppersful three times a day.

Capsules or tablets: These may contain powdered root or leaves. Take 1 or 2 capsules or tablets up to three times a day.

Of course, echinacea should not be considered a substitute for other medical interventions in rapidly accelerating infections. If an infection persists or worsens, seek medical advice. Many serious medical conditions are not appropriate for self-diagnosis or self-medication and require the supervision of qualified health care providers. Always use caution when practicing self-care.

Even if you do catch a cold, echinacea may help you to shake it off sooner than you otherwise might. During a period of infection, when the body is running low on resources, echinacea has been found to have a strong and direct force on the body's ability to speed healing. In other words, when you're in bed with a cold, your body can use all the help it can get. In that case, says Varro Tyler, Ph.D, professor emeritus at the Purdue University School of Pharmacy in West Lafayette, Indiana, echinacea "may result in clear improvements."

Tackling the Flu

The same holds true for flu. In one study conducted in Germany, liquid echinacea extract was shown to help ease the symptoms of influenza and speed recovery. Another study, this one reported in 1978, found that echinacea root was significantly effective in attacking influenza viruses. Another clinical study, in 1992, found that volunteers who took echinacea showed marked resistance to flu viruses. And volunteers who took echinacea, but who still came down with the flu, exhibited far fewer symptoms than untreated patients.

Peter Thiess, who founded a large pharmaceutical herb company in Germany, says he's had great success using echinacea to fight off flu.

"I used to be very susceptible to flu when I was under a lot of stress," says Thiess, author of *The Family Herbal.* "Almost every time I needed to prepare for an important business trip and had to work around the clock to get ready, I would experience various symptoms such as head congestion, fever blisters on the lips, feverish chills, or that general 'down' feeling."

Today, he says, with the help of echinacea tincture, "I can handle intense periods of stress very well without being forced by my immune system to slow down or curtail my activities."

Getting What You Pay for

When purchasing echinacea, stick to brand names you trust. Because echinacea and other herbs are not federally regulated, consumers can't always be certain that what they're buying is a pharmaceutical grade of echinacea—or even if the product contains any echinacea at all. How to tell? Good-quality echinacea products produce a harmless tingling sensation in the tongue. Your best chance of getting the right amount of echinacea lies in choosing products from well-established suppliers.

GLUCOSAMINE SULFATE FOR OSTEOARTHRITIS

Here's how Helen, a 52-year-old office manager, describes the arthritis in her knees: "It's so painful," she says, "that I won't stand up unless you put a gun to my head." If misery loves company, Helen has plenty of both. Arthritis, in its many forms, is the leading cause of disability in the United States. More than 40 million Americans have it, including 23 million women and a quarter million children. Each year, the disease costs $60 billion in medical care. The various types of arthritis comprise the number-one medical problem in the world. More people suffer from arthritis than from cancer, heart disease, and AIDS combined. But because arthritis is not a fatal disease, it doesn't always garner the attention it merits. While a variety of drugs are used to help ease the discomfort of arthritis, many can produce serious side effects in patients. But new research suggests that a natural supplement called glucosamine sulfate not only blunts arthritis pain as effectively as conventional medicines but may even help to reverse the disease.

Arthritis is actually a catch-all term that refers to more than 100 conditions. The most common form of the disease, and the one we'll focus on here, is called osteoarthritis. (Indeed, it is this form of arthritis that most people are referring to when they talk about arthritis.) Osteoarthritis afflicts more than 16 million Americans, men and women alike. Arthritis can be a minor annoyance or a disabling disease that takes over every aspect of your life.

Symptoms of osteoarthritis usually don't appear until you're in your 40s or 50s. Most people over the age of 60, in fact, would show some signs of arthritis on X rays, although only a third will experience symptoms. Some health experts estimate that as many as 90 percent of us will get some form of osteoarthritis at some point in our lives.

Osteoarthritis occurs as a result of the breakdown of the cartilage in the joints. In a normal joint, the ends of the bones are covered with cartilage, a durable, elastic tissue that protects the bones and allows the joint to move freely. Cartilage gets the oxygen and nutrients it needs by absorbing them, like a sponge, from the joint fluid (called synovial fluid). As the joint bends, waste products are squeezed out of the cartilage; as the joint relaxes, nutrients and oxygen are absorbed. (Controlled movement, therefore, benefits the joints.)

In osteoarthritis, the cartilage thins out and may even wear away, leaving areas where bones rub directly against each other. As a result, the edges of the bones may thicken and form bony swellings called spurs (medically known as osteophytes). Stiffness and dull pain in the joints, with little or no inflammation, are generally the result. These are the typical symptoms of osteoarthritis.

The weight-bearing joints (hips, knees, and spine) are most frequently involved in osteoarthritis. Other joints often affected are the finger joints closest to the tips of the fingers, which may develop bony knobs. The joint at the base of the thumb and the big-toe joint may also be affected. Osteoarthritis rarely affects the wrists, elbows, shoulders, ankles, or jaw. While osteoarthritis may affect more than one joint at a time, the disease does not affect other systems or organs of the body.

Glucosamine at a Glance

Description: Glucosamine is a modified sugar molecule that your body makes from glucose (blood sugar).

Function: Glucosamine is a building block for substances called mucopolysaccharides (MPS), which

Osteoarthritis is considered a chronic disease, but it may not necessarily get progressively worse, and many people with the condition are relatively free of symptoms. Few people are severely disabled by the disease.

What Causes Osteoarthritis?

While a breakdown of the cartilage in the joints is essentially the source of the symptoms of osteoarthritis, it is not always clear why this breakdown occurs. Most often, the thinning of the cartilage is attributed to years of wear and tear and the inability of the body to repair the resulting damage. Previous injury that causes inflammation in a joint can also make it more likely to be affected by osteoarthritis. Unusual stress on a joint, either through a repetitive activity, such as typing or playing a sport, or because of excess body weight, may bring about the changes associated with osteoarthritis, per-

are important for development of cartilage, bone, ligaments, nails, hair, and skin. Glucosamine also stimulates connective tissue, encouraging it to repair itself.

Action: Glucosamine sulfate supplements appear to help reduce osteoarthritis pain by helping the body protect—and perhaps rebuild—cartilage.

haps earlier than is typical. Some individuals are born with a misalignment of their joints that leaves them prone to osteoarthritis. And in some cases, there appears to be a genetic component.

Diagnosing Arthritis

Diagnosing osteoarthritis can be difficult, partly because the disease's symptoms may be mistaken for those of other conditions, including injuries, muscle or spinal-disc problems, or even other forms of arthritis. X rays and laboratory tests can help rule out other conditions. But perhaps the most valuable diagnostic tool available to doctors is the physical examination, including a medical history and a detailed discussion of the symptoms.

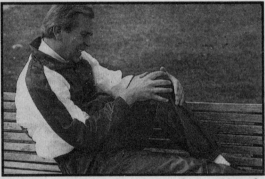

Weight-bearing joints such as the knee are frequent targets of osteoarthritis.

To help your doctor make a diagnosis, be prepared to tell him or her which part of your body hurts; what the pain feels like, when it began, and how long it lasts; what, if anything, seems to trigger the pain or make it worse; when and if you have stiffness or other symptoms; what activities you may have trouble doing; and what, if anything, helps to relieve your pain.

Conventional Relief

The best conventional treatment for osteoarthritis generally involves prescribed exercises to keep the joints flexible, encourage nourishment of the cartilage, and strengthen the surrounding tissues; joint protection, often based on the suggestions of a physical or occupational therapist, to limit further damage; and, when necessary, both drug and nondrug measures to ease discomfort and decrease stiffness. Losing excess weight, eating a nutritionally balanced diet, and getting enough rest are also often part of the treatment prescription.

As noted previously, it is the movement of a joint that forces oxygen and nutrients into the cartilage and removes waste products, thus helping to keep the cartilage healthy. When the pain and stiffness of arthritis set in, however, moving the affected joint is the last thing on many patients' minds. The tendency to limit the motion of an affected joint can actually aggravate the problem and may lead to even greater loss of mobility. While excessive or very strenuous activity may not be appropriate, gentle range-of-motion exercises can actually decrease stiffness and pain. Range-of-motion exercises are used to put a joint through the full range of its natural motion without excessive stress. They are essential to any treatment plan for arthritis. Your doctor or a physical therapist can show you appropriate exercises or recommend an exercise class designed for people with arthritis.

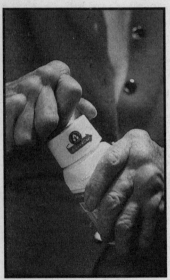

Special caps can make pill bottles easier for arthritic fingers to open.

Extremely important, too, is protecting arthritic joints from injury or excessive strain. This may boil down to simple techniques such as using your forearm, rather than your bent wrist and hand, to push open a door or placing heavy kitchen equipment on shelves at waist height. Increasing knowledge of the needs of people with arthritis has also led to an abundance of products designed to make daily tasks easier on painful joints. For example, forks, spoons, knives, and other utensils with soft, built-up handles that make gripping easier are now available in many grocery and department stores. Even if your joints aren't currently painful enough to affect your grasping ability, such joint-friendly devices can limit strain and may help prevent progression of symptoms.

Additional measures to help ease the pain and stiffness of arthritis include heat and cold treatments. Hot showers or baths or heating pads may improve flexibility, especially before exercise or other physical activity. And cold packs can often help numb a particularly painful joint.

If these measures don't give adequate pain relief, your doctor may recommend medication. Most often, it will be acetaminophen or a nonsteroidal anti-inflammatory drug (NSAID). Some NSAIDs, such as aspirin, ibuprofen, and naproxen sodium, are available over the counter. Stronger NSAIDs, such as sulindac, indomethacin, tolmetin sodium, and fenoprofen calcium, are available only by prescription. These medications can be quite effective in relieving joint pain. As with many other drugs, however, they can have some uncomfortable and even dangerous side effects, especially if you must take them on an ongoing basis.

Arnold Fox, M.D., who augments his conventional practice with alternative medicine in Beverly Hills, California, avoids prescription arthritis drugs whenever possible.

"When I was a young medical student, I dreamed of saving the world with these and other drugs," Fox says. "But as I began treating patients, saw the effects of these powerful chemicals on the human body, I began to doubt the wisdom of relying too heavily on drugs."

It's not that pharmaceuticals aren't effective, Fox says. They are. But sometimes they can cause more problems than they solve.

Aspirin and other NSAIDs, for example, may irritate the stomach lining and cause severe internal bleeding in some people. Taken in large amounts over the long term, they can also cause kidney and liver damage. Some research even suggests that these drugs may actually inhibit cartilage repair and increase the progression of the disease.

"I use conventional medications when necessary but work to get my patients off of them as soon as possible," says Fox.

Is Surgery for You?

If medications don't work to relieve your symptoms, or if your disease is severe, your doctor may recommend surgery to ease your pain. There are two main types of operations for arthritis.

The first is "clean-up" surgery to repair a damaged joint by removing debris, correcting a deformity, or fusing bones. In the second type of surgery, the arthritic joint is removed and replaced with an artificial one.

Both operations have improved the lives of thousands of arthritis victims. But Fox is among the physicians who view surgery as a last-ditch effort.

"Frankly, I'm scared of surgery," Fox concedes. "In many cases, it can work wonders. But there is no such thing as a safe surgery. Every single surgery is a risky procedure. Your body is undergoing trauma, your breathing and other vital functions are taken over by machines, body tissue and organs are being cut and stitched, and foreign objects and fluids are being introduced. All it takes is a small misstep or a moment of lost concentration, and disaster can strike. And even if the surgery does go off without a hitch, there may be complications."

If Fox eschews pharmaceutical medicines and surgery, what's left? Glucosamine. It's Fox's first line of defense.

What Is Glucosamine?

Glucosamine is a modified sugar molecule the body makes from glucose (blood sugar). Our bodies need glucosamine to function properly. That's because glucosamine is a kind of building block for substances called mucopolysaccharides (MPS), which are important for the development of cartilage, bone, ligaments, nails, hair, and skin. Glucosamine stimulates connective tissue, encouraging it to repair itself.

Think of glucosamine as a security guard whose mission it is to protect the tiny biochemical factories in your body called chondrocytes. Found largely in joints, chondrocytes produce collagen and other substances and assemble them into cartilage. Normally, glucosamine is on the job to see that orders are filled. But if you have arthritis, your chondrocytes cannot produce enough glucosamine, and degeneration results.

The chondrocytes begin to act as if they are under orders to destroy cartilage. And the "factory" just can't make enough new cartilage to replace what's lost. In severe joint damage, chondrocytes stop making glucosamine altogether.

But there's considerable evidence that taking glucosamine supplements can prompt your body to flip a "switch," convincing the haywire chondrocytes to stop destroying cartilage—and even begin to rebuild it.

How Glucosamine Works

Just how glucosamine convinces chondrocytes to stopping running amok is unclear.

What we do know from animal studies is that glucosamine works nothing like aspirin or other NSAIDs. Instead, it appears to function as a nutrient.

Most of the initial research on glucosamine was conducted in Europe, where pharmaceutical companies were quick to realize the nutrient's importance in treating arthritis. In fact, glucosamine sulfate has become the arthritis treatment of choice for many European physicians, who turn to conventional drugs only when glucosamine sulfate proves to be ineffective.

Throughout Portugal, for example, it's glucosamine you'll receive if your doctor hands you a diagnosis of arthritis. In 1982, more than 250 Portuguese doctors participated in a nationwide study to determine the supplement's effectiveness in treating arthritis. The physicians gave 1,506 osteoarthritis patients a daily dose of 1,500 milligrams of glucosamine sulfate for six to eight weeks. In another group, 1,077 arthritis sufferers were treated with NSAIDs, such as ibuprofen, or with corticosteroids. At the end of the trial, 95 percent of patients in the glucosamine group showed marked improvement, compared to 70 percent of patients in the NSAIDs group. Consequently, the Portuguese doctors, as a group, rated glucosamine a better arthritis treatment than standard drugs.

Scores of other tests also suggest that glucosamine sulfate may be a valuable nutrient for arthritis patients. In one trial, Philippine researchers at the National Orthopedic Hospital in Manila studied 20 people with arthritis. Each subject was about 60 years old and suffered from osteoarthritis of the knees. Half the subjects were given 1,500 milligrams a day of glucosamine. The other group was given a placebo (sugar pill). Eight weeks later, the glucosamine group reported significant reductions in joint pain, swelling, and tenderness.

Is Glucosamine Safe?

To date, human studies have shown no toxicity from supplements of glucosamine sulfate. And in animal studies, glucosamine was found to be 1,000 to 4,000 times safer than indomethacin, a common NSAID

In another experiment, scientists at Vigevano General Hospital in Pavia, Italy, studied 80 arthritis patients for 30 days. The subjects, all in their 60s, were suffering from osteoarthritis of the neck, lumbar (lower) spine, or multiple joints, conditions that doctors find most difficult to treat. Half the patients were given a daily dose of 1,500 milligrams of glucosamine sulfate; the other half got a sugar pill. At the end of the trial, ten patients in the glucosamine group reported that their symptoms had disappeared. No one in the control group made such a claim.

Buoyed by the results of such experiments, more and more researchers have been testing glucosamine sulfate. Among the more well-known studies:

• Researchers gave 24 patients with osteoarthritis of the knee either 500 milligrams of glucosamine sulfate three times a day or a placebo. In six to eight weeks, those who received the supplement enjoyed significant re-

used to relieve osteoarthritis pain. Other animal studies have detected no toxic effects of glucosamine, even after animals consumed the human equivalent of one-third of a pound of glucosamine every day for more than a year. For humans, that would be like taking several full bottles of glucosamine every day.

ductions in pain, joint tenderness, and swelling. They reported no side effects.

- Eighty osteoarthritis patients suffering from pain, swelling, and restricted movement were given either glucosamine sulfate or a placebo. After three weeks, 73 percent of patients in the glucosamine group reported marked improvement of symptoms. Scientists biopsied (surgically removed and examined a small amount of tissue) cartilage taken from the glucosamine patients, moreover, and found that the tissue appeared far healthier than samples taken from the placebo group.

- In 1994, researchers at several clinics in Germany and Italy set out to determine the effectiveness of glucosamine sulfate. The test group was composed of 141 patients with osteoarthritis of the knee. One group received a placebo. The other got 1,500 milligrams a day of glucosamine sulfate. After four weeks, 55 percent of glucosamine-taking patients noted improvements, compared to 38 percent in the placebo group.

Glucosamine or Pharmaceuticals?

One of the first glucosamine sulfate studies compared the nutrient's effectiveness with that of conventional painkillers. In 1980, researchers at the First Medical Division in Venice, Italy, studied 30 elderly patients with advanced osteoarthritis. For three weeks, half the patients were given injections and pills of glucosamine sulfate; the other half received injections and pills of a standard painkiller.

At the end of the trial, both groups reported significant decrease in joint pain and improvement in joint function. But after all treatments were stopped, the glucosamine subjects continued to note improvements, but the control subjects did not. Four patients in the glucosamine-treated group, in fact, became symptom free, but none in the control group did.

Thus, the researchers concluded, even in cases of severe degenerative joint disease, glucosamine sulfate reduces pain as well as painkilling pharmaceutical drugs.

Two years later, researchers at St. John's Hospital in Oporto, Portugal, compared glucosamine sulfate to ibuprofen. For eight weeks, 40 patients with osteoarthritis of the knees took daily doses of either 1,500 milligrams of glucosamine or 1,200 milligrams of ibuprofen. In the first two weeks, ibuprofen seemed to relieve pain faster and better than glucosamine sulfate. But after two more weeks, no more improvements were reported by the ibuprofen camp. At the end of eight weeks, patients in the glucosamine group were reporting far less pain than those in the ibuprofen group and showed more significant improvements in joint function.

Another study comparing the two drugs followed 200 patients with osteoarthritis of the knees for four weeks. As in the previous study, one group got 1,500 milligrams of glucosamine a day; the other received daily doses of 1,200 milligrams of ibuprofen. After one week, ibuprofen takers were feeling better than glucosamine patients. But by the second week, and notably by the fourth week, glucosamine patients said they felt just as good as ibuprofen patients. More important, researchers noted, 35 percent of people taking ibuprofen reported experiencing side effects, including nausea, itching, and fatigue. Only six percent of glucosamine patients reported mild stomach upset. Seven subjects had to stop taking ibuprofen because of toxicity; only one person in the glucosamine group had to pull out of the study.

Prescription for Glucosamine

Take 1,500 milligrams of glucosamine sulfate a day until arthritis symptoms have decreased. Then reduce the dosage to 1,000 milligrams a day for two weeks. As your symptoms continue to improve, reduce the

The researchers concluded that glucosamine sulfate was, in some ways, more effective than conventional pain relievers in treating osteoarthritis patients. But, they noted, it could take two to three weeks of glucosamine therapy before a patient notices results.

What to Take

Glucosamine is found to some degree in most of the foods we eat, especially fish and meat. But no food is particularly rich in the nutrient, and most glucosamine appears to be destroyed by cooking.

That means you need to take glucosamine supplements to achieve medical benefits. Glucosamine is available in three varieties: glucosamine sulfate, glucosamine hydrochloride, and N-acetylglucosamine (NAG). Which should you take?

dosage to 500 milligrams a day. If your symptoms disappear, stop taking the supplement. If symptoms return or worsen, simply increase the dosage. You should begin to notice improvements by two weeks and definitely by eight weeks.

Some holistic practitioners insist that all three varieties of glucosamine are equally effective in relieving arthritis pain. However, studies in humans have focused primarily on glucosamine sulfate. Further testing of the other varieties as well as comparisons of the three are needed in order to assess the benefits of glucosamine hydrochloride and NAG.

Likewise, the usefulness of glucosamine sulfate preparations that also contain chondroitins is

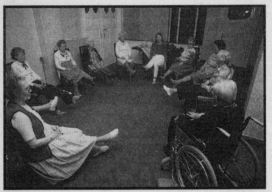

Exercises to keep joints flexible are essential to any arthritis treatment plan.

yet unclear. (Chondroitin is produced by the body and helps cartilage retain fluid, keeping it spongy.) Nearly all the research in Europe has used glucosamine sulfate supplements alone, not in combination with chondroitins.

For individuals who need to restrict their sodium intake, glucosamine sulfate is available in a potassium-bound form; look for glucosamine sulfate potassium chloride.

A final important note is that even if you take glucosamine sulfate, it would be extremely wise to also take lifestyle steps to protect your joints. That means eating a nutritious diet, getting regular exercise and rest, keeping excess weight off, and, if possible, refraining from repetitive motions that put excessive stress on your joints.

Can Glucosamine Reverse Symptoms?

In Europe, long-term studies are being done to determine whether the supplement may actually reverse damage caused by osteoarthritis. It takes three to five years before X rays and other tools can detect reversal, so the jury is still out.

In one completed study, samples obtained by scanning electron microscopy showed that cartilage taken from subjects who had used glucosamine sulfate appeared healthy and young.

If you suffer from arthritis, ask a holistically oriented physician whether glucosamine might help you. It's possible that you and your doctor can come up with a therapy to reduce your symptoms, and perhaps even reverse them, without the risk of dangerous side effects.

Mint, Chamomile & Ginger for Sour Stomachs

There's a reason that bowl of peppermints awaits you as you leave a restaurant. Peppermint has a cherished history as an herb that soothes your stomach after a big meal. The same goes for ginger. When you were a child, your mother may have given you ginger ale when your tummy was upset. If it was made from real ginger extract, it likely did a world of good. Research shows that ginger is a potent antinausea medicine. And if your parents are from Europe, your mom probably brewed you a cup of chamomile tea to ease stomach pain and help you to relax.

As more of us turn to natural medicines, we're discovering that there's a good deal of evidence to support using the home remedies our mothers and grandmothers gave us when we were sick. Remember the story of Peter Rabbit? After his harrowing adventure in the farmer's garden, Peter's mother fixed him a nice cup of chamomile tea to settle his nerves and queasy stomach. Today, most herbal researchers would applaud Mrs. Rabbit's homespun medical intervention.

"Chamomile is one of the few medicinal plants that still have a prominent role in traditional medicine," says Daniel B. Mowrey, Ph.D., director of the American Phytotherapy Research Laboratory in Salt Lake City, Utah. "And peppermint is probably our best-known remedy for stomach problems."

In Asian and West Indian countries, ginger is the remedy of choice when stomachs growl and complain. The pungent, spicy herb, moreover, is at its best when used to treat motion sickness. Some studies, in fact, indicate that ginger may be a better remedy than conventional over-the-counter and prescription treatments.

The best thing about all three herbs is that most, if not all, are in your kitchen now or are readily available. That's good news when it comes to stomach complaints, which are among the most common human ailments.

Why Do Stomachs Hurt?

There's probably no one on earth who has not suffered from an upset stomach at one time or another. Stomachaches rank right up there with headaches and colds. It seems we're always coming down with them.

Any of a number of factors can aggravate our digestive systems. Our stomachs may gripe if we eat rich foods, foods to which we are unaccustomed, poorly prepared foods, heavily fried foods, foods that have been contaminated by bacteria and other germs — or just too much food.

Stress also contributes to various stomach disorders. Ever eat when you were upset or worried about something? Your tummy may have awakened you that night to express its concerns as well.

It's a good thing our stomachs are well designed. We use them all the time. Digestive enzymes in

Mint at a Glance

Peppermint
Latin name: *Mentha piperita*

Spearmint
Latin name: *Mentha spicata*

Description: Peppermint and spearmint once were considered to be the same plant. Both have square stems and are invasive perennials, which send up new

the mouth begin to break down food into nutrients that our bodies can use. After food is swallowed and passes through the esophagus, it empties into the stomach, a saclike organ that connects the esophagus to the small intestine. Like a bagpipe, the stomach is flexible. It can expand or collapse.

The walls of your stomach consist of layers of muscle lined with special glandular cells that secrete gastric juices. These juices continue the digestive process that began in your mouth, breaking food up into useful nutrients and waste products.

Your stomach is packed with blood vessels and nerves. The upper part of the stomach is called the fundus. The strong muscle at the lower end of the stomach forms a ring called the pyloric

plants from spreading roots. Mint species are difficult to differentiate because they interbreed. Mints produce tiny purple, pink, or white flowers that appear in July and August. Their leaves are fragrant and toothed.

Habitat: Peppermint and spearmint are native to Europe and Asia. There are other types of mint native to South Africa, America, and Australia. Peppermint and spearmint have been naturalized throughout North America from southern Canada to Mexico.

sphincter, which controls the passage of food from the stomach to the small intestine.

The stomach has one primary function—to digest food. Gastric glands begin secreting juices the moment you see or even mention food. Once that food hits your stomach, even more activity takes place. Gastric juices contain enzymes, hydrochloric acid, and mucus. Hydrochloric acid and enzymes, such as pepsin and lipase, begin the process of breaking food down into its constituent parts. Pepsin begins to digest proteins; lipase starts to break down fats. Gastric juices also contain a substance that facilitates absorption of vitamin B_{12} in the small intestine. And mucus is important because it protects the stomach wall from the acid's caustic actions and from abrasion by food particles.

The only substances absorbed from your stomach are water and some types of sugar. The rest are absorbed in the intestine.

Your stomach muscles create a churning action that mixes food with gastric juices, forming a pastelike mixture called chyme. At regular intervals, the stomach contracts, and the pyloric valve relaxes, squirting an amount of chyme into the small intestine.

The small intestine has three main parts. The first ten inches or so is called the duodenum.

The second part, which is some eight feet long when uncurled, is the jejunum. And the last eleven feet or so is called the ileum.

When the chyme reaches the duodenum, it is mixed with powerful enzymes secreted by the pancreas and with bile secreted by the gallbladder. The enzymes further break down proteins and carbohydrates and the bile breaks down fats so that these nutrients can be absorbed through the intestinal wall and into the bloodstream and lymphatic channels. Also present in the small intestine are alkalis, which help to neutralize the acids from the stomach and protect the intestinal lining.

Finally, the waste products from the digestion process proceed to the large intestine, or colon. There, excess water is absorbed and the waste material is stored until it can be voided from the body through the anus.

Along this digestive way, however, things can go wrong. One of those things is called heartburn.

Heartburn

Heartburn's main symptom is a burning sensation in the chest, just behind the breastbone, or sternum. You also may feel a burning in your throat, caused by acid backing up into the esophagus. Symptoms of heartburn generally occur soon after you've eaten something too fast, you've laid down too soon after eating, or you've eaten a type of food that simply doesn't agree with you. Discomfort may last a few minutes or several hours.

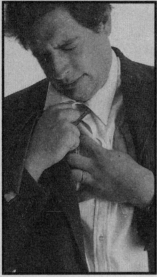
Heartburn results when stomach acid backs up into the esophagus.

What causes heartburn is a lower esophageal sphincter (a valve-like ring of muscles) that isn't closing as tightly as it should. Certain foods contain chemicals that relax the sphincter and encourage it to open when it shouldn't. These include tomatoes, citrus, garlic, onions, chocolate, coffee, and alcohol. You can also get heartburn if there's too much food in your stomach or too much pressure on your stomach muscles.

Indigestion

There are many theories about what causes indigestion, but no one knows for sure. Heavily fried foods, for example, seem to cause indigestion in some people. Symptoms may include excess gas, belching, abdominal pressure or pain, mild nausea, or vomiting.

As we grow older, our digestive systems gradually become less efficient. Thus, our stomachs may have a harder time handling the load if we drink or eat too much or misuse analgesics, such as aspirin, that can cause digestive upsets.

If the strain is too much, our stomachs may decide to empty themselves. That queasy feeling you get before you throw up is called nausea. Although it's usually caused by a digestive problem or an infection, such as food poisoning, nausea can result from hormonal and other imbalances during pregnancy or from motion sickness.

Don't Rock the Boat

If you don't get seasick, you probably know somebody who does. Sickness resulting from motion, such as that produced by a boat, car, or plane, is a common malady. Gail, who lives in Deerfield Beach, Florida, had a miserable time on a Caribbean cruise she took with her husband. "I've never felt so sick in my life," she recalls. "It was all I could do to lift my head."

Motion sickness occurs when your brain receives conflicting information from your sensory organs. Your eyes may not be detecting motion to the same degree as the balance mechanism in your inner ear. Your central nervous system, not quite knowing what to do, reacts to the stressful phenomenon by activating the nausea center in your brain.

Your first line of defense for treating heartburn, indigestion, or nausea caused by motion sickness, pregnancy, or any other reason, may be to try any of a number of over-the-counter remedies that are readily available (although, if you are pregnant, be sure to check with your doctor before trying any over-the-counter medication).

Pharmaceutical Fixes

To alleviate the symptoms of heartburn and indigestion, many people turn to over-the-counter antacids, which contain substances that absorb excess acids. While these work on heartburn quickly, their effect is temporary. Also available for heartburn relief are the H_2blockers such as ranitidine (Zantac), famotidine (Pepcid), cimetidine (Tagamet), and nizatidine (Axid). These medications decrease the production of stomach acid. Originally available only by prescription, lower dosages of these medications have recently become available over the counter. They do not act as quickly as antacids, but they provide longer lasting relief.

For people with heartburn that does not respond to over-the-counter treatments and who experience heartburn more than twice a week, a doctor visit is generally in order. The doctor may prescribe higher doses of H_2blockers, which appear to be helpful in at least 60 percent of patients. Although uncommon, side effects from high-dose H_2blockers may include sleepiness, fatigue, headache, dizziness, constipation, or diarrhea. Treatment with these higher doses also requires monitoring by the doctor.

If the high doses of H_2blockers don't do the trick, the doctor may prescribe one of the proton pump inhibitors (PPIs), such as omeprazole (Prilosec) or lansoprazole (Prevacid). They, too, inhibit the production of stomach acid, but not in the same way as the H_2blockers. You may need to take these daily, and there is some concern about harmful effects to the stomach lining and tumor formation from long-term use.

For motion sickness, over-the-counter remedies such as the antihistamine dimenhydrinate (Dramamine), which reduces the sensitivity of the motion-detecting nerves in your ear, may help. Scopolamine, which is available in a time-released skin patch, may reduce the muscle spasms and contractions that trigger vomiting.

Worn behind the ear, the patch pumps medicine into the bloodstream. Also an option is the sea band, which is a bracelet worn on the wrist; the bracelet stimulates acupressure points that alleviate nausea.

If the pharmaceutical products available for digestive problems don't appeal to you, you may find surprisingly effective relief from chamomile, mint, or ginger. All three are effective in reducing the symptoms that accompany many digestive disorders.

Mint's Other Uses

Mint long has been an ingredient of candies and savory foods. It's also an effective anesthetic. Menthol, the main component of peppermint, is found in many pain-relieving skin creams, including Solarcaine, Unguentine, Ben-Gay, and Noxzema Medicated Cream.

Prescription for Mint

Tea: Steep 1 to 2 teaspoons of mint leaves in one cup of boiling water in a covered container for 20 minutes. Drink two or more cups a day.

Marvelous Mint

Mint is one of the most reliable home remedies for an upset stomach. Grandmas have been handing out mints for centuries to treat indigestion, flatulence, and colic. The two types of mint you're most likely to encounter are spearmint and peppermint. Although they once were considered the same plant, peppermint actually is a natural hybrid of spearmint. It's also the more potent of the herbs.

Menthol also relieves nasal, sinus, and chest congestion and is an ingredient in Mentholatum and Vicks VapoRub.

In laboratory tests, peppermint oil has killed several strains of bacteria as well as the herpes simplex virus, which causes cold sores and genital herpes.

Tincture: Take 1 teaspoon of the solution up to three times a day.

Peppermint owes part of its healing power to an aromatic oil called menthol. Spearmint's primary active constituent is a similar but weaker chemical called carvone.

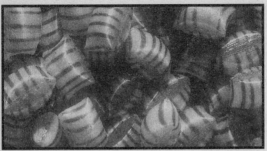

After-dinner mints can actually aid digestion.

Oil of peppermint contains up to 78 percent menthol. Menthol encourages bile (a fluid secreted by the liver) to flow into the duodenum, where it promotes digestion. Menthol also is a potent antispasmodic; in other words, it calms the action of muscles, particularly those of the digestive system.

Menthol's medicinal value has been borne out in numerous studies with animals and with humans. German and Russian studies show that peppermint not only helps to stimulate bile secretion but also may prevent stomach ulcers. The potent oil is also capable of killing myriad microorganisms that are associated with digestive and other problems. Recent studies, moreover, suggest that menthol may be useful in treating irritable bowel syndrome, a common but hard-to-treat digestive disorder in which the bowel contracts, causing a crampy type of adult colic.

Comforting Chamomile

Chamomile's medicinal secret is the volatile oil derived from its daisy-like flowers. An extract produced from the herb can reduce muscle spasms and inflammation of mucous membranes, making it a useful treatment for indigestion and menstrual cramps. Chamomile also contains chemicals that fight infections that cause minor illnesses.

Several studies indicate that chamomile is a good digestive aid. The herb contains a wide variety of active constituents. Bisabolol, one of its prime constituents, has anti-inflammatory properties and relaxes the smooth muscle lining of the digestive tract. In experimentally induced gastritis and other inflammations of the mucous membranes, chamomile consistently demonstrated quick and prolonged anti-inflammatory effects.

As long ago as 1914, researchers were publishing papers proclaiming the herb's ability to block the actions of convulsants and other chemicals that cause spasms. Chamomile's sedating properties were documented in the

1950s. But we're still learning just how the herb works.

For years, researchers attributed the herb's antispasmodic effect to the presence of flavonoids, such as apigenin and luteolin. But several recent trials have demonstrated that other constituents also contribute substantially to the herb's total sedative action. The importance of chamazulene and its precursor, matricin, has been demonstrated in nearly all of chamomile's actions.

Chamomile at a Glance

German chamomile
Latin name: *Matricaria recutita*

Roman chamomile
Latin name: *Chamaemelum nobile*

Description: German chamomile is an erect annual. Roman chamomile is a low-growing perennial. Both

Prescription for Chamomile

Tea: Steep 2 to 3 teaspoons of chamomile flowers in one cup of boiling water in a covered container for 15 to 20 minutes. Drink up to three cups a day.

The anti-inflammatory constituents of chamomile, including azulene, chamazulene, bisabolol, and matricin, appear to have distinct modes of action. Some of them are more powerful than others but perform for a shorter period of time; others are milder but perform for longer periods of time.

What we're learning now is that apparently all of chamomile's constituents must work together for the herb to function medicinally. Thus,

plants produce flowers that look like daisies and have a remarkable fresh apple scent. Both plants have feathery leaves. The plants flower from late spring through late summer.

Habitat: Both chamomiles are native to Europe, Africa, and Asia. They have been naturalized in North America and are widely cultivated.

Tincture: Use ½ to 1 teaspoon up to three times a day for nervousness, indigestion, or menstrual cramps.

Essential oil: Take 1 to 3 drops three times a day.

chamomile would seem to be one of the plant kingdom's best examples of holistic medicine at work.

Chamomile may also help to prevent and heal ulcers. In one study, two groups of animals were fed a chemical known to cause ulcers. Animals that were also given chamomile developed significantly fewer ulcers than those who did not receive it. And animals that did develop ulcers recovered more quickly if they were fed chamomile.

In 1979, experiments verified chamomile's protective healing effects on the mucous membranes of the gastrointestinal tract. In the first experimental studies, chamomile inhibited formation of ulcers produced under several condi-

---

Chamomile's Other Uses

In Spain, chamomile has long been used as a flavoring for sherry. Chamomile is also an ingredient of some skin-care products and shampoos, especially for blondes.

In Europe, chamomile is one of the best-selling herbal teas. As a medicinal, chamomile is used by one German pharmaceutical company in a product called Kamillosan, which is used to treat wounds, inflammations, indigestion, and ulcers.

---

tions, including stress and administration of drugs, such as alcohol.

Although the ultimate role of hydrochloric acid in naturally occurring ulcers is a subject of dispute, it has been shown that chamomile is able to inhibit formation of ulcers that are experimentally induced by that acid.

If you plan to try chamomile medicinally, make sure you get as much of the volatile oil as possible, says pharmacognosist Varro Tyler, Ph.D., professor emeritus at the Purdue University School of Pharmacy in Indiana. Many of the chemicals contained in the oil are lost through steam when tea is brewed. Even a very strong tea may contain only a small percentage of chamomile's volatile oils. So steep your tea in a

---

Because of its well-known sedating properties, chamomile may be used as a mild tranquilizer. In addition, the herb is an infection fighter. Chamomile extracts seem especially good at killing the yeast fungus *candida albicans*.

In a study with rabbits, chamomile stabilized impaired kidney function in the animals. And when it was given to arthritic rats, the herb's essential oil markedly reduced inflammation.

---

covered container. You could also try eating the chamomille flowers after you've brewed your tea instead of simply throwing them in the trash or garden.

Ginger at a Glance

Latin name: *Zingiber officinale*

Description: Ginger is a tropical perennial that grows from an aromatic tuber that is knotty and buff colored. Ginger flowers rarely in cultivation. In the

Prescription for Ginger

Ginger tea, candied ginger, and authentic ginger ale (made with real ginger) all will help your stomach to feel better. But encapsulated ginger powder is thought to be the most effective way to use the herb in treating digestive disorders. That's because you can take more ginger without experiencing discomfort. Raw ginger or powder can burn the palate.

"The biggest mistake people make is not taking enough ginger," says herbalist Daniel B. Mowrey. "If you don't taste a little ginger on your breath or in your throat about five minutes after swallowing the capsules, you haven't taken enough."

Rejuvenating Ginger

Ginger is another well-documented remedy for stomach disorders. Ginger appears to reduce inflammation in a similar way to nonsteroidal anti-

---

wild, it produces dense, conelike spikes. Its leaves are grasslike.

Habitat: Ginger's origin is uncertain, but some botanists think it probably is native to India and southern China. Ginger has been introduced to other tropical areas, including the West Indies and Florida, where it is cultivated.

For severe motion sickness, take four 400 milligram ginger capsules 20 minutes before your journey. For mild to moderate cases, take two capsules 15 minutes before traveling. In mild and severe cases, take two to four ginger capsules the minute you begin to feel nauseated.

To make ginger tea, pour one pint of boiling water over one ounce of ginger root powder or large slices of fresh ginger root, and simmer up to 20 minutes. A strong cup of ginger tea contains about 250 milligrams of the herb. A heavily spiced ginger dish contains about 500 milligrams. The amount in real ginger ale varies considerably.

inflammatory drugs (NSAIDs), such as aspirin and ibuprofen; it slows associated biochemical pathways. Ginger is also a mild stimulant that promotes circulation.

Ginger's root contains chemicals called gingerols and shogaols, which relax the intestinal tract, preventing motion sickness and relieving the nausea, vomiting, colicky stomach cramps, and diarrhea that often accompany stomach flu.

The herb has been studied thoroughly as a remedy for motion sickness. The British medical

Ginger's Other Uses

Ginger is a staple of Chinese, Japanese, Southeast Asian, East Indian, West Indian, and North African cooking. It helps to spice up beverages, fruit salads, meats, poultry, fish, preserves, pickles, sweet potatoes, carrots, beets, pumpkins, peaches, puddings, breads, muffins, cakes, and cookies.

Ginger also appears to be a good remedy for treating a variety of disorders. The herb, for example, has a 40 to 50 percent success rate in treating dizziness.

Ginger is also effective at lowering cholesterol. An oleoresin of ginger root included in a high-cholesterol diet was capable of preventing a rise in cholesterol in control animals. It is thought that the herb interferes with the cholesterol absorption process.

journal *Lancet,* for example, reported in 1982 that ginger is a "very effective" motion sickness medicine.

Several studies show that two or three ginger capsules taken one half hour before a trip and two to three capsules taken at one to two hour intervals during a trip are effective in preventing motion sickness.

Nausea that is caused by motion sickness is a complex reaction involving various areas of the brain as well as the digestive tract. Although it's

---

By reducing blood platelet clumping (the process involved in clotting), ginger may reduce the risk of heart attack or stroke. In experiments with rats, oil of ginger inhibited clumping of the blood cell components.

As an antispasmodic, ginger is helpful in reducing menstrual cramps. Researchers also have found that ginger helps to kill some forms of influenza virus.

Indian studies show that ginger increases the immune system's ability to fight infection. And studies have confirmed the herb's anti-inflammatory effects, leading to speculation that it might be useful in treating arthritis.

In addition, ginger helps to lower blood pressure. And in animal experiments, the herb has demonstrated an ability to shrink some tumors.

---

unclear exactly how ginger works, it appears to act directly on both the stomach and the brain. For that reason, ginger may be used to relieve dozens of ailments, including any form of nausea, gas, heartburn, flatulence, diarrhea, and vertigo (dizziness). The *Lancet* journal article recommends ginger capsules, ginger tea, or ginger ale for morning sickness associated with pregnancy. And a few conventional physicians are prescribing ginger for patients who become nauseated after having cancer chemotherapy treatments.

Is Mint Safe?

There have been no toxic effects reported from normal consumption of mint. But the sharp, pungent fragrance of concentrated mint oils may cause gagging in some people.

Is Chamomile Safe?

Most people experience no problems after consuming chamomile. But because its flowers contain pollen, a tea made from the herb may cause dermatitis or other allergic reactions in a small number of people. If you are highly sensitive to ragweed, chrysanthemums, or other members of the botanical Compositae family, use chamomile with discretion.

Ginger has demonstrated a success rate of 75 percent in curing morning sickness and stomach flu. Research in animals suggests that extracts of fresh ginger may inhibit gastric secretions and perhaps play a role in preventing some gastric ulcers.

Is Ginger Safe?

For most people, ginger is perfectly safe for consumption. Some people who have used it for motion sickness have reported symptoms of heartburn.

Ginger does have a long history as an herb that can promote menstruation, so if you are pregnant, you may want to err on the safe side and limit your consumption to two cups of ginger tea per day.

GINKGO &
ALZHEIMER DISEASE

*Maria, a social services agency worker in her 40s, was
beginning to forget things: a friend's birthday, a
luncheon appointment, the last place she
had left her car keys. After reading a
magazine article about herbal
medicine, Maria decided to try
ginkgo biloba, which Chinese
doctors have been using for
thousands of years to boost cerebral
(brain) function. To Maria's surprise,
her short-term memory improved.
Even more surprising, she seemed able to
think more clearly than she had in years.*

Ginkgo may not make you smarter. But several
studies indicate that this ancient Asian herb
does improve cerebral function and may prove
to be a valuable natural remedy for treating the
symptoms of Alzheimer disease, a devastating
illness that erases the memory and personality

of its victims. "Ginkgo can be useful for treating the dementia associated with Alzheimer's," says medical botanist James Duke, Ph.D., former chief of the U.S. Department of Agriculture's Medicinal Plant Laboratory. "And because ginkgo increases blood circulation in the brain, it can help in many types of cerebral disorders."

The U.S. Food and Drug Administration does not recognize ginkgo as a medicine. But, "research on ginkgo and Alzheimer's is producing extremely good results in France and Germany," says Daniel B. Mowrey, Ph.D., director of the American Phytotherapy Research Lab in Salt Lake City, Utah.

Europeans have been using ginkgo extract for years to ward off Alzheimer disease and other cerebral disorders associated with aging, including forgetfulness; mild confusion; ringing in the ears; and inability to concentrate. In some countries, ginkgo is a registered drug, among the most commonly prescribed for organic brain disorders. In lower doses, ginkgo is sold over the counter in many European countries.

In France, for example, ginkgo accounts for four percent of all prescription medicines. And the herb comprises one percent of prescription sales in Germany, where it is licensed for treatment of "cerebral insufficiency" and used to treat problems ranging from impaired memory, dizziness, and tinnitus (ringing in the ears) to headaches, nervousness, and anxiety.

Although ginkgo is among the better-studied herbs, more trials need to be conducted before U.S. physicians are likely to prescribe the herb on a routine basis. Still, many scientists are hopeful that ginkgo may one day yield a drug that can prevent or treat the dread Alzheimer disease, for which there currently is no cure.

What Is Alzheimer Disease?

Alzheimer disease afflicts more than four million Americans. Among its victims is former President Ronald Reagan. Although the disease may strike younger people, most Alzheimer victims are over the age of 65. And the number of those affected is likely to climb as the baby boomers hit their later years. By the middle of the next century, some statisticians warn, Alzheimer will afflict as many as 14 million Americans.

Imagine losing your soul. That's what doctors say it's like to have Alzheimer disease. The fatal disease is marked by progressive degeneration of brain tissue, which leads to devastating mental decline and the onset of dementia. Victims forget where they live, what they had for breakfast. How many times have you read in your local newspaper about an elderly Alzheimer victim who has wandered away in the middle of the night and then forgotten how to get home? Most sufferers ultimately lose the ability to recognize the faces of the people who love them.

Alzheimer disease slowly strips victims of their intellectual functions, including the ability to concentrate, comprehend ideas, and retain new information. Speech deteriorates, attention strays, simple calculations become increasingly difficult to perform. Understandably, Alzheimer victims often feel frustrated and bewildered.

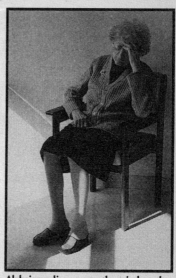

It's not surprising, then, that the agitation and anxiety suffered by Alzheimer patients is frequently expressed in severe mood swings, depression, paranoia, and even violent behavior. People with Alzheimer disease may experience moments of extreme selfishness, exhibit childish behavior, and have an increased tendency to misplace things. They may also

Alzheimer disease saps the minds and memories of its victims.

demonstrate physical symptoms, such as impaired equilibrium (balance) or an odd gait.

Eventually, Alzheimer patients may lose the ability to communicate at all or become incontinent or otherwise physically helpless.

There is no cure for Alzheimer disease. If you get it, it will change forever the lives of the loved ones who care for you. The disease may run its course from insidious onset to death in just a few years. Or, it may play out, agonizingly, for more than 20. Most patients with Alzheimer disease survive about seven years after diagnosis.

For American adults age 65 and older, Alzheimer disease is among the top ten leading causes of death. Nearly half of those over the age of 85 suffer from the disease.

Until recently, researchers thought that whites were four times more susceptible to developing

Ginkgo at a Glance

Latin name: *Ginkgo biloba*

Description: Ginkgo is a stately tree that can grow up to 100 feet tall and attain a girth of 20 feet. It produces fan-shaped leaves with two lobes. Female

Alzheimer disease than blacks. But a new study—the first major study of the disease in ethnic groups—shows that blacks and hispanics are at far greater risk than nonhispanic whites.

Even blacks who do not have a gene commonly linked to Alzheimer disease are four times more likely to develop the disease by age 90 than white nonhispanics. The increased rate among blacks and hispanics was present even after researchers took into account the patients' sex, family histories, and educational levels.

The findings surprised the researchers, who now speculate that the ethnic groups may develop Alzheimer disease for a variety of reasons, genetic and environmental.

"This is the first major study that has shown an increased risk of Alzheimer's in these ethnic populations," says Dr. Neil Buckholz, chief of the Dementias of Aging Branch at the National

ginkgo trees produce apricot-size, orange fruits, whose seeds may be eaten. But the fruits are messy and foul smelling.

Habitat: Ginkgos are native to Asia but are cultivated widely on streets and in yards throughout much of the United States.

Institute on Aging, which funded the study published in March 1998 in the *Journal of the American Medical Association.* (*JAMA*) "It raises some interesting questions and is the beginning to getting some answers."

We used to call this debilitating condition senility, and it was accepted as a normal consequence of aging. Now we recognize that Alzheimer is a devastating crippler. But why do some people get it, and others don't?

What Causes Alzheimer Disease?

The gradual loss of brain function associated with Alzheimer disease seems to result from nerve damage incurred when tangles of an abnormal insoluble protein called amyloid invade the areas of the brain that govern thought and memory. Because no treatment can halt the progression of this tangling, victims eventually sink into a shadow world they cannot comprehend.

Scientists can't say just what causes the tangling to occur. A few years ago, some researchers speculated that Alzheimer disease might be triggered if people ingested minute particles of aluminum deposited in food from cookware or present in antacids, deodorants, and canned foods and beverages.

Another theory links brain plaques with free radicals—unstable, molecules that can produce destructive chemical reactions in the body. Both theories are controversial and unproved.

In a minority of cases, trauma appears to contribute to the onset of Alzheimer disease. About 15 percent of Alzheimer victims have a history of head injury.

It is most likely that Alzheimer disease results from a combination of faulty genes and environmental factors.

It's in the Genes

Researchers have identified three genes that are associated with early onset of Alzheimer disease. For many Alzheimer patients, however, it's a fourth gene, apolipoprotein-E, or ApoE-4, that appears to do the dirty work.

ApoEs are normally occurring blood proteins (lipoproteins) required for transport of fatty substances in the body. They are among the lipoproteins that carry cholesterol in the blood, which may get deposited in blood vessel walls. The kind of ApoE you have is genetically determined. Among whites, the presence of ApoE-4 is associated with higher Alzheimer risk. This finding also suggests that there may be a link between Alzheimer disease and the clogging of arteries that results in strokes and heart attacks.

Scientists originally assumed that ApoE-4 was the culprit behind Alzheimer in all ethnic groups. But the recent study of blacks and hispanics suggests that other genetic or environmental factors increase the likelihood of developing Alzheimer in those minority populations, says Richard Mayeux, M.D., a professor of neurology, psychiatry, and public health at Columbia University College of Physicians and Surgeons in New York.

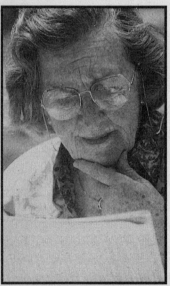

The brain needs a healthy flow of blood to function at its best.

For five years, Mayeux and colleagues followed 1,079 Medicare recipients of different ethnic backgrounds in the Washington Heights neighborhood of northern Manhattan. At the beginning of the study, none of the volunteers had Alzheimer disease. During annual physical and neurological examinations, researchers were able to track those who went on to develop the disease—221 people—and those who did not.

What the researchers discovered was that ApoE-4—the gene they thought had caused the disease—could not be blamed for the increased rates of Alzheimer disease in blacks and hispanics. Even without that gene, those minority groups got Alzheimer disease at higher rates than whites who have the gene. The next step, the researchers say, is to identify the genes or other factors that account for the disparity.

"We need to know what those other risk factors are," says George Martin, M.D., a neuropathologist at the University of Washington in Seattle. "If African Americans and Hispanics have some unidentified genes that put them at further risk, we need to know what they are and how they work, so we can target therapy for them."

How the genes are involved is a mystery. Perhaps certain forms of ApoE cause destruction of nerve cells in the brain. It's also possible that the protein, working in combination with other substances, is involved in formation of plaques.

At any rate, it seems a certainty that genes play a role in the development of Alzheimer disease. If your father or mother had Alzheimer, you run a higher risk of getting the disease.

What Doctors Can Do

No drug available today can halt the onslaught of Alzheimer disease. No therapy can reverse the damage done by the disease. But some drugs can slow the progression of the disease to a degree—if it is caught early. Other drugs may help to control mood swings and other behavioral problems associated with Alzheimer.

In 1993, the FDA approved the first drug for treatment of Alzheimer disease. It is called tacrine hydrochloride, and in clinical tests, it has delayed progression of the disease by six months and improved mental function in people whose disease was not far advanced. The drawback is that the drug may cause liver problems. People who take it must be monitored weekly to ensure that their livers are functioning properly.

A more recent entrant into the medication marketplace is a drug called donepezil hydrochloride (Aricept TM). It, too, appears to slow the progression of the disease when given to those with mild to moderate deterioration and it does so without damaging the liver. However, donezepil's beneficial effects may lessen as the disease progresses. It can also cause uncomfortable side effects such as nausea, vomiting, diarrhea, insomnia, muscle cramps, fatigue, anorexia, headache, and dizziness.

In addition, several drugs are prescribed to treat specific symptoms of the disease: haloperidol (Haldol) and thioridazine (Mellaril) for aggressive behavior and agitation; sertraline (Zoloft) for depression; and zolpidem (Ambien) and diphenhydramine for insomnia.

Can Ginkgo Help?

Ginkgo is among the most studied plant medicines in Europe and the United States. Ginkgo's benefits seem to derive from its ability to improve circulation in virtually every area of the body, especially the brain. Ginkgo opens up blood vessels and keeps them supple, thus helping to prevent circulatory problems and enhance the body's ability to nourish itself.

Ginkgo also helps to fight free radicals, those highly reactive molecules that result from our body's use of oxygen. Researchers think free radicals probably play a role in degenerative diseases, such as cancer and Alzheimer, and in the aging process itself. Antioxidants such as ginkgo scavenge free radicals, reacting with them and leaving harmless molecules in their place.

And ginkgo has the ability to interfere with a bodily substance called platelet activation factor (PAF). Discovered in 1972, PAF is involved in

(Continued on page 154)

Ginkgo's Other Uses

Ginkgo isn't just used to treat Alzheimer disease and other cerebral disorders. The herb appears to have myriad uses.

In Germany, ginkgo extract has been approved as a supplemental treatment for certain kinds of hearing loss, leg cramps, and numbness caused by poor circulation.

Ginkgo also appears to improve blood flow to the heart muscle and may be useful for preventing heart attacks by reducing the risk of internal blood clots.

A study published in the *Journal of Urology* indicates that ginkgo may relieve impotence caused by the narrowing of arteries that supply blood to the penis. Sixty men with erection problems caused by impeded penile blood flow were given daily doses of 60 milligrams of ginkgo. After six months of treatment, 50 percent of the subjects were able to achieve erections and 45 percent of the remaining subjects showed improvement.

In a French study, ginkgo significantly improved the vision of people suffering from macular degeneration, the leading cause of adult blindness. Gingko appears to prevent destruction of the retina, a nerve-rich area in the eye.

Ginkgo may also be of use in preventing and treating strokes, the third-leading cause of death in the United

States. As we grow older, blood flow to the brain decreases, resulting in less food and oxygen for brain cells. Ginkgo significantly increases blood flow to the brain and may speed recovery from some types of stroke (it shouldn't be used for strokes due to bleeding, or hemorrhagic strokes).

Ginkgo also appears to benefit certain forms of hearing problems. A French study showed significant recovery among people who took ginkgo to treat cochlear deafness, which is caused by decreased blood flow to nerves responsible for hearing. And a 13-month study of 103 people who suffered from tinnitus, persistent ringing in the ears, found that ginkgo conclusively reduced symptoms.

Another study in animals found that ginkgo extract may help to prevent kidney and liver damage caused by cyclosporin A, an immunosuppressive drug used in transplants. Ginkgo was found to be as effective as vitamin E and glutathione in protecting against such damage.

Blood clots also seem to be positively affected by ginkgo. In 1992, German scientists administered 240 milligrams of ginkgo extract a day to 20 patients suffering from various diseases that led to dangerous blood clotting. After 12 weeks, clotting factors had decreased in every one of the patients. The researchers reported in the medical journal *Fortschrift Medizine* that ginkgo "can positively influence these cardiovascular risk factors over the long term."

a staggering number of biological processes, including asthma attacks, arterial blood flow, and formation of blood clots that can lead to heart attacks and strokes. By inhibiting PAF, ginkgo may keep us from developing many of the diseases that strike as we grow older.

The most important ginkgo studies relate to its use in preventing, treating, or influencing vascular diseases, brain function, impotency, inflammation, and asthma.

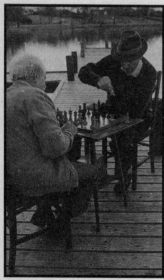

A standardized extract from ginkgo leaves seems to significantly improve blood flow, especially in medium-size and small arteries. In elderly subjects, the extract alleviated dizziness and loss of memory, probably by allowing more blood to get to the brain.

Ginkgo may enhance an Alzheimer patient's ability to concentrate.

Thus, ginkgo may be useful in treating Alzheimer disease, especially if the disease is diagnosed early. "It seems that the earlier you catch [diagnose] the disease, the greater the chance that you can reverse it by taking ginkgo extract," says herbalist Mowrey.

Among the early symptoms that ginkgo may alleviate are deterioration of the short-term memory, depression, absent-mindedness, anxiety, dizziness, inability to concentrate, mental confusion, and tinnitus.

In October 1997, *JAMA* published results of a multicenter study indicating that ginkgo extract may be of "significant benefit" in treating dementia associated with Alzheimer disease. The double-blind study (meaning neither researchers nor subjects knew who was getting the active substance and who was simply getting a sugar pill) was designed to investigate the effects of standardized ginkgo extract on 309 patients with mild to severe dementia associated either with Alzheimer disease or a condition known as multi-infarct dementia (in which areas of impaired circulation result in tissue death in the brain). For 52 weeks, patients were treated with either a placebo or 40 milligrams of ginkgo extract taken three times a day. At the end of the trial, patients were given standardized tests to measure cognitive impairment, social behavior, and general psychopathology. The researchers reported that 27 percent of patients who received 26 or more weeks of ginkgo treatment scored at least four points higher on the 70-point Alzheimer Disease Assessment Scale–Cognitive Subscale (ADAS–Cog), compared with 14 percent who did as well in the placebo (sugar pill) group. In assessments of daily living skills and social behavior, 37 percent of ginkgo patients showed improvement, compared with 23 per-

Disastrous Results

We know more about ginkgo than we do about many herbs—thanks in large part to a natural disaster.

In 1963, a typhoon damaged many of the ginkgo trees in Sendai, Japan, where Koji Nakanishi was studying four of ginkgo's chemical compounds: ginkgolides A, B, C, and M.

The best way to study ginkgolides is to obtain them from the bark of the tree's root. But usually the bark cannot be harvested without destroying the trees, many of which can live to be 1,000 years old.

Because so many ginkgos were uprooted by the storm, Nakanishi and colleagues were able to obtain a large quantity of roots. This helped them to make significant advances in understanding the structure of ginkgolides, which they presented in a paper in Stockholm in 1966.

Ginkgo's medical benefits depend on a proper balance of two active components: ginkgo flavone glycosides and terpene lactones. The combined actions of the

cent of those who took placebos. The overall condition of 40 percent of placebo takers worsened during the study, compared with only 19 percent of those taking ginkgo.

Moreover, the researchers said, "Adverse events [side effects] associated with (ginkgo) were no

constituents are stronger than those produced by each alone.

Flavone glycosides are substances found in many plants and fruits, especially citrus. The chemicals are potent antioxidants that scavenge free radicals, highly volatile molecules that can damage many parts of our bodies. Flavonoids also protect cells against the breakdown of arachidonic acid, an unsaturated fatty acid that keeps cell membranes healthy and permeable. Bioflavonoids such as those found in ginkgo protect blood vessels.

Terpene lactones are found in ginkgo in the form of bilobalides and ginkgolides. Terpene lactones offset processes that lead to formation of blood clots. Ginkgo's terpene lactones improve circulation in the brain and other parts of the body by bringing oxygen to tissues and enhancing absorption of glucose (blood sugar) by body tissues. Terpene lactones, as well as other constituents of gingko, also protect nerve cells from damage during periods of oxygen deprivation that can lead to strokes.

different from those associated with the placebo."

JAMA termed the results "particularly promising" in light of the fact that no satisfactory treatment now exists for management of Alzheimer.

The ginkgo used in the study was a concentrated leaf extract standardized to 24 percent ginkgo flavone glycosides and 6 percent terpene lactones, the same extract widely used in Europe for treatment of cognitive disorders. This extract is available in the United States under a variety of trade names (check labels).

Similarly encouraging were results of a ginkgo study published recently in the journal *Phytomedicine*. The double-blind, placebo-controlled, randomized study investigated the effects of ginkgo extract in 156 patients with Alzheimer disease or multi-infarct dementia. After 24 weeks, 28 percent of patients who took ginkgo extract achieved consistently higher test scores,

Prescription for Ginkgo

Alzheimer disease: Consult your physician before giving ginkgo to anyone with Alzheimer disease. Most Alzheimer studies have used 240 milligrams of ginkgo extract a day.

compared with only 10 percent in the placebo group.

In another study, 31 patients with mild to moderate memory impairment were given a standardized ginkgo extract and observed for six months. The extract, as in earlier tests, contained 24 percent flavonoid glycosides and 6 percent terpenes. At the end of the trial, researchers reported that ginkgo clearly had a "beneficial effect on mental efficiency" in the elderly Alzheimer patients.

One of the most famous ginkgo studies of aging-induced cerebral disorders was reported in 1986 by the French medical journal *La Presse Médicale*. Researchers developed a scale of 17 items to evaluate 166 geriatric patients in several centers. Markers included vivacity, short-term memory, disturbances in orientation, anxiety, depression, emotional stability, initiative, cooperation, sociability, personal care, ability to walk, appetite, vertigo (dizziness), fatigue, headache, sleep, and

To improve cerebral function: Take 40 milligrams of ginkgo three times a day. Look for capsules containing 24 percent ginkgo flavone glycosides and 6 percent terpene lactones. It may take four to six weeks before you see results.

tinnitus. After taking ginkgo extract for three months, the subjects improved in every area, and they continued to improve over time.

A 1996 study in Germany focused on 216 patients with mild to moderate symptoms of Alzheimer. The patients were divided into two groups. For one month, patients in the first group were treated daily with standardized ginkgo extract. Patients in the second group received a placebo. At the end of the trial, the subjects were tested for mental, behavioral, and motor skills. Those who had taken ginkgo showed great increases in mental alertness and improvement in mood. But little improvement was noted among patients in the placebo group.

And in a study of eight women, short-term memory and reaction time improved dramatically after they had taken ginkgo.

Is Ginkgo Safe?

Ginkgo is considered to be safe for most people if taken in moderate amounts. If you take extremely large amounts, you may experience irritability, restlessness, diarrhea, nausea, and vomiting. In addition, you may want to start with a small dose of the extract and gradually increase it to full strength to

How Does
Ginkgo Compare?

Those are the success stories. There are failures, too. In some studies, ginkgo has not proved to be more effective than conventional drugs in treating several symptoms associated with Alzheimer disease. But because ginkgo produces no serious side effects, and no problems have been observed from interactions, the herb may be preferable to drugs in many instances.

Of course, you should never attempt to treat Alzheimer or any serious disease on your own. If a loved one is suffering from Alzheimer, discuss ginkgo with the patient's physician. The doctor may decide to give ginkgo a try, since no current therapies are successful in truly alleviating Alzheimer disease. Using ginkgo certainly won't hurt. In fact, it just might help.

avoid the headache and dizziness that can occur at the start of gingko therapy. People taking warfarin (Coumadin) or using aspirin on a regular basis may want to avoid also taking standardized gingko extract, since their blood-thinning action may be increased. Never attempt to treat yourself with ginkgo or any herb or supplement without first consulting your physician.

SAW PALMETTO
FOR ENLARGED
PROSTATE

Paul, a production manager from Plantation, Florida, watched his father suffer the progressive symptoms of prostate enlargement, a benign (noncancerous) condition that affects most men in one form or another as they grow older. When Paul turned 45, the age at which many men begin to develop prostate problems, he decided to take precautions. He went to a local health-food store and bought a bottle of saw palmetto berry extract.

"Now I take saw palmetto every day," Paul says. "I don't want to have to go through what my father went through."

Here's what you can expect if you develop the problems Paul's father faced. You wake once, twice, maybe even three times during the night with an urgent need to urinate. But, you find it difficult to empty your bladder. If this sounds familiar, you may have an enlarged prostate.

If it's any consolation, you're by no means alone. Most men over the age of 60—and many in their 50s—develop some symptoms associated with benign prostatic hyperplasia (also called hypertrophy), or BPH. The condition is so common that some physicians consider it a normal consequence of aging in males.

Left untreated, BPH may get progressively worse. And it can lead to potentially dangerous complications, including bladder and kidney infections.

It wasn't so long ago that men simply had to suffer through the symptoms of prostate enlargement, which can range from mild to severe. Or they were forced to undergo complicated surgery to have their prostates resectioned or removed.

Today, there are prescription drugs that can help to shrink your prostate or ameliorate the symptoms associated with the condition. And if you do require surgery, there are less-invasive procedures that can save you time and pain.

But there's also a natural remedy that more men are trying these days. It's an extract made from the berries of the common saw palmetto plant. The jury's still out on the clinical effectiveness of this herbal cure, but the research that's been conducted in this country and in Europe looks promising. In the meantime, more physicians are recommending saw palmetto as a natural alternative treatment. And more men like Paul are giving it a try.

What Is Saw Palmetto?

Driving south along Interstate 95, through Georgia and Florida, you should have no problem spotting the saw palmetto, a shrubby plant whose daggerlike fronds are arranged in a fan shape.

For centuries, the Indians in these parts have prized the saw palmetto. They ate the berries as food and used the leaves to weave baskets and thatch huts. In addition, tribal healers valued saw palmetto berries as a potent medicine for a multitude of ailments, in particular, those that plague men as they grow older.

Saw Palmetto at a Glance

Latin name: *Serenoa repens*

Description: Saw palmetto is a low, shrubby palm with a creeping, branchy stem. Leaves are wide, green, and deeply divided. Flowers are inconspicuous and appear on a branched cluster, followed by purple fruit.

Today, like echinacea, another herbal gift from indigenous Americans, saw palmetto has found its way to cities across the United States. From New York to Los Angeles, it's not uncommon to see men in business suits purchasing bottles of the herbal remedy in pharmacies and health-food stores.

Like Paul, they've probably read articles in newspapers and magazines touting saw palmetto's ability to prevent and treat prostate enlargement, a condition that's become almost synonymous with so-called male menopause.

Until recently, most conventional physicians knew nothing about saw palmetto's medicinal uses. Now, more are beginning to express an interest in the herb, says Alan R. Gaby, M.D., former president of the American Holistic Medical Association.

Habitat: A native of North America, saw palmetto is found on coastal plains from Florida and Texas to South Carolina. The plant prefers swampy, low-lying land.

"I recommend saw palmetto berry extract for many men with enlarged prostate glands," Gaby says. "Studies have shown that it can improve urinary flow rates and reduce symptoms like urinary hesitancy and weak flow. In many cases, it works as well or better than prescription drugs—and its cheaper and safer."

What Is
Prostate Enlargement?

The prostate is a walnut-shaped gland located just below a man's bladder. The gland surrounds a portion of the urethra, the narrow tube through which urine exits the body. The prostate's primary function is to produce an essential portion of the seminal fluid that carries sperm. And, through the action of an enzyme called 5-alpha-reductase, the prostate converts testosterone into dihydrotestosterone (DHT), a powerful hormone that spurs prostate cells to multiply.

The benign growth of the prostate appears to be a normal part of the aging process in men. At puberty, the gland grows as a boy matures. Then, until the age of 45 or so, the prostate stays about the same size. Why the prostate once again begins to grow starting in middle age is as yet unclear.

Prostate enlargement can block the urethra, creating difficulties with urination. This may occur either as a result of tissue actually blocking the urethra or of pressure from the prostate on the urethra itself.

What Are the Symptoms?

If your prostate becomes enlarged, you may experience symptoms that range from mildly annoying to severely painful. One of the first signs is a frequent, urgent need to urinate. Once you try to do so, however, you may produce a weak or intermittent stream and find yourself straining, dribbling, or unable to completely empty your bladder.

Such symptoms are especially common and troubling when they occur at night. Many men who have an enlarged prostate have to get up several times each night to urinate. Not only is this inconvenient, it's exhausting, and some men subsequently must be treated for anxiety and sleep disorders.

Eventually, lingering pools of urine in the bladder may become sites of infection or stone formation. If the outflow of urine becomes completely blocked, urine within the bladder may back up to the kidneys, leading to permanent damage of those organs; inability to urinate is a medical emergency that requires immediate professional treatment.

What Your Doctor Can Do

Just a few years ago, the only solution for treating an enlarged prostate gland was painful invasive surgery to reduce the size of the prostate or remove it altogether. Today, there are several new and more comfortable treatment options, from hormone-blocking drugs to lasers that can remove prostatic tissue without your having to be hospitalized.

The prescription medication finasteride (Proscar) has shown some ability to gradually reduce prostate size and lessen symptoms. Proscar is a 5-alpha-reductase inhibitor, meaning it blocks this enzyme, thus decreasing the production of DHT. With less DHT available to spur prostate growth, the rate of enlargement

Measuring Urine Flow

Men over 50 routinely are given a urinary flow test—a quick, inexpensive way to measure their prostate function. The subject urinates in a funnel, which drains into a beaker attached to a computerized scale. A readout of the urinary flow gives the peak flow rate per thousand, followed by average flow and total

slows. It may take up to six months, however, before beneficial effects are noticed.

Proscar also decreases the level of a protein called prostate specific antigen (PSA). PSA levels are often elevated in men who have prostate cancer, and measurement of PSA is a common screening test used to detect prostate cancer. The concern is that Proscar, by decreasing the level of PSA, might mask the presence of prostate cancer. Doctors can adjust for this effect when they measure the level of PSA in a patient on Proscar. However, in order to do this, they must obtain a baseline PSA measurement before the patient begins taking Proscar.

Another group of prescription medications that are used to treat BPH are the alpha-1-adrenergic blockers, including terazosin (Hytrin), prazosin (Minipress), doxazosin (Cardura), and tamsulosin (Flomax). These medications relax

volume expelled. In addition, the test measures one of the characteristics of benign prostatic hyperplasia: dribbling.

Healthy peak urinary flow ranges from 35 to 50 milliliters per second. As the prostate enlarges and obstructs the bladder, the urinary flow rate generally declines.

the smooth muscle tissue of the prostate, the neck of the bladder, and the urethra. Originally, this class of medications was used to treat high blood pressure. Indeed, Hytrin, Minipress, and Cardura are often good choices for men who suffer from both high blood pressure and symptoms of BPH. Unlike its chemical cousins, Flomax does not generally have a significant blood–pressure-lowering effect; it has been marketed, from its introduction, as a treatment for the symptoms of BPH.

Another Natural Remedy

In Germany, where physicians routinely prescribe saw palmetto extract to reduce enlarged prostates, men who suffer from the condition are also finding relief with another herbal extract made from the root of stinging nettle *(Urtica dioica)*.

Although most Americans have never heard of it, stinging nettle extract has been used safely and effectively in Germany and other European countries for more than a decade. Several studies, in fact, show that the herbal extract can reduce symptoms of benign prostatic hyperplasia by as much as 86 percent after only three months of therapy.

One study found that after eight weeks of treatment with a daily dose of four capsules of stinging nettle extract, 82 to 100 percent of symptoms plaguing men with BPH were reduced.

None of these prescription medications improves BPH in all cases, and none is without side effects. Proscar, for example, can cause a decrease in sex drive, impotence, and a decrease in the volume of ejaculate. And women who are or who could become pregnant should not take or handle Proscar and should avoid contact with the semen of a man who is taking Proscar; there is the potential for genital abnormalities in a male fetus as a result of a pregnant woman's exposure to the drug.

Another study found that patients suffering from abnormal proliferation of prostate cells, a condition that can lead to prostate cancer, reported an 86 percent improvement in symptoms after three months of treatment with a standardized stinging nettle extract.

How does stinging nettle work? That's what researchers at St. Luke's Roosevelt Hospital in New York set out to determine in 1995. The scientists concluded that the extract inhibits binding of a testosterone-related protein to its receptor site on prostate cell membranes.

Some herbal remedy manufacturers have combined stinging nettle with saw palmetto and the extract from another herb called pygeum, which has traditionally been used to treat urinary problems. The formula could provide a safe and effective treatment for reducing enlarged prostates. Unfortunately, however, the supply of pygeum is at risk due to overharvesting.

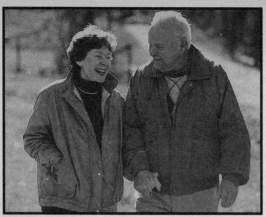

BPH appears to be a normal part of the aging process in men.
Hytrin, Minipress, and Cardura can cause orthostatic hypotension (dizziness that occurs when rising from a sitting or lying position), especially early on in treatment. They may also cause fatigue, nasal congestion, general dizziness, insomnia, headache, and a decrease in the volume of ejaculate. Flomax may cause abnormal ejaculation, dizziness, and nasal stuffiness.

What About Surgery?

If your prostate is severely enlarged or you have very uncomfortable symptoms that have not responded to medication, your doctor may recommend that you have an operation.

Surgical techniques provide relief from BPH symptoms in about 85 percent of patients who have them. With the most common type of surgery, the patient is given a regional anesthetic, but the surgeon makes no incision. Instead, a small instrument called a resectoscope is passed through the penis into the prostate by way of the urethra. Using an electrical apparatus at the end of the scope, the surgeon carves away the inner prostate, leaving a hollow shell through which urine can flow. This procedure is known as transurethral resection of the prostate, or TURP.

About 15 percent of men who undergo TURP experience complications, which may include urinary incontinence or impotence. Some patients experience infection or bleeding. And others require a second operation to reopen the urinary tract.

Several kinds of laser resectors have been used on an outpatient basis with good results. Again, the instrument is passed through the urethra to the prostate. The laser is then fired, and the resulting heat quickly vaporizes excess prostate tissue.

There is also a device called the Prostatron, which uses microwaves to heat the gland and destroy excess tissue. Procedures using this device, however, are not as widely available as are others.

If none of these operations works, your doctor may recommend removal of your prostate gland. Naturally, this should be considered a last resort.

In the meantime, you may want to ask your physician about saw palmetto. Certainly, taking an herbal supplement is easier and more convenient than using a medicine with side effects or undergoing surgery, however safe the procedure. The question is: Does the clinical evidence support saw palmetto's growing popularity as an alternative medicine for enlarged prostates?

What Is Saw Palmetto?

Although it is native to the United States, saw palmetto, like other alternative medicines, first became popular in Europe, where herbal remedies are big sellers. In many European coun-

Saw Palmetto's Other Uses

Saw palmetto has a folk history as a treatment for disorders of the urinary and reproductive systems. The berries once were brewed to make an aphrodisiac. Men have used the herb at times to boost sperm count. And some women have tried saw palmetto to increase breast size, although there is no evidence to substantiate the practice.

tries, several prescription and over-the-counter remedies for prostate enlargement are based on saw palmetto extract. In Germany, for example, saw palmetto is an approved drug often recommended by physicians.

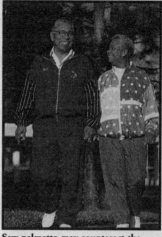

Saw palmetto may counteract the hormones causing prostate growth.

In the United States, however, saw palmetto's reputation is not well established. Although more physicians are considering use of the herb— Paul's doctor, for example, urged him to try it— the Food and Drug Administration (FDA) says

Saw palmetto has expectorant (bringing up phlegm), nutritive, and sedative (relaxing) properties. The herb's fruits have a mildly stimulating action on the respiratory and genitourinary systems. For that reason, saw palmetto has been used to treat chronic and acute bronchitis and severe chest congestion.

There are some anecdotal reports that saw palmetto may be used to treat atrophy (wasting) of the testicles, but no evidence backs this claim.

the scientific evidence supporting saw palmetto is scant and has restricted manufacturers' marketing claims. But many naturopathic physicians and herb experts in this country disagree.

"Studies in Europe show that an extract from saw palmetto berries appears to counteract the effects of certain male sex hormones, called androgens, that may cause prostate enlargement. It also has an anti-inflammatory activity" says pharmacognosist Varro E. Tyler, Ph.D., professor emeritus at Purdue University School of Pharmacy in Indiana.

In Belgium, for example, researchers gave saw palmetto extract to 505 men with benign prostate disease. At the end of the trial, the researchers concluded that saw palmetto had aided urinary flow, reduced residual urinary volume and prostate size, and otherwise improved the patients' quality of life. Saw palmetto, moreover, began to produce results

Prescription for Saw Palmetto

Capsules: Herbalists commonly recommend a daily dose of 320 milligrams of an oil-based saw palmetto extract to shrink an enlarged prostate gland and provide relief of symptoms. This often works out to two capsules a day, one in the morning and one in the

within 45 days. Proscar, on the other hand, can take six months to a year to work, if indeed it works at all.

After 90 days of saw palmetto treatment, 88 percent of patients and their physicians said they considered the therapy to be effective. Said the Belgian researchers: "The extract of saw palmetto appears to be an effective and well-tolerated pharmacologic agent in treating urinary problems accompanying benign prostate hypertrophy."

Just how saw palmetto achieves results remains unclear. Studies in mice have shown that an extract of saw palmetto berries inhibits the enzyme 5-alpha-reductase. That's the chemical, you'll recall, that spurs production of DHT, which causes prostate tissue growth. Saw palmetto extract also appears to inhibit DHT from binding to cell receptor sites. This increases the breakdown of DHT and encourages its excretion.

evening (but check the label on the product you buy just to be sure).

If saw palmetto alone fails to work, some herbalists recommend combining saw palmetto extract with an herb called pygeum. The dose of pygeum generally recommended is 1 to 1½ teaspoons of tincture three times a day.

In a subsequent human trial, 80 percent of men with benign prostate enlargement reported significant improvement in symptoms after using saw palmetto extract.

But not all the studies of saw palmetto have been as encouraging. In one double-blind trial, 110 patients took either a placebo or an extract of saw palmetto for one month. The patients who received saw palmetto showed statistical improvement, but not enough for the researchers to conclude that saw palmetto was an effective treatment.

Another study, this one of 32 patients for 7 to 30 months, produced similar results. Patients did show improvement, but the evidence to support saw palmetto's use as a medicine was considered to be inconclusive.

Researchers got the same results in a third trial, a randomized, double-blind study of 30 patients

Is Saw Palmetto Safe?

Taken as directed, saw palmetto is safe to consume. Detailed toxicology studies carried out on mice, rats, and dogs have shown that the herb has no toxic side effects. Be sure, however, to inform your health care practitioner that you are taking saw palmetto.

suffering from prostate adenoma (noncancerous tumor). The scientists found that saw palmetto extract gave patients some relief. But again, the gains were considered only minimal.

How Does Saw Palmetto Compare?

But there's enough clinical evidence for medical botanist James Duke, Ph.D., to support the use of saw palmetto. "Saw palmetto is every bit as good as its pharmaceutical alternatives for treating the symptoms of enlarged prostate and even shrinking the gland," says Duke, former chief of the U.S. Department of Agriculture's Medicinal Plant Laboratory.

At the Whitaker Wellness Institute, Inc., in Newport Beach, California, founding physician Julian Whitaker, M.D., frequently prescribes saw palmetto for men with prostate problems.

"The fat-soluble extract of saw palmetto berries is much more effective than Proscar, and saw palmetto costs one fourth the cost of Proscar," Whitaker says.

Proscar costs most men about $75 a month. A comparable amount of saw palmetto extract costs less than $50 a month and in some areas as little as $15.

Moreover, Whitaker says, "Proscar is effective in less than 50 percent of cases after patients have taken it for a full year. Saw palmetto extract is effective in nearly 90 percent of patients, usually after four to six weeks."

Nonetheless, it's unlikely that you'll see saw palmetto as a federally approved drug any time soon.

In 1990, a company called Enzymatic Therapy petitioned the FDA to have saw palmetto approved for treatment of BPH. The federal agency rejected the application. FDA officials said that they recognized results of clinical trials that showed "statistically significant" improvements in men who took the herbal extract. But the FDA concluded that such data was not "clinically significant."

Meanwhile, Merck, which manufactures Proscar, predicts that annual sales will soon top $1 billion.

What Should You Take?

So where does that leave you if you're suffering from symptoms of prostate enlargement? The first thing to do is to see your doctor to rule out other conditions, including prostate cancer. Then the two of you can determine whether it would be in your best interest to try prescription medications, saw palmetto extract, or a combination.

When purchasing saw palmetto, be sure to buy an extract standardized to contain 85 to 95 percent fatty acids and sterols. Berries alone, although cheaper than the extract, would have to be taken in much greater amounts to achieve beneficial effects. Only standardized fatty acid sterols have been studied for their ability to shrink prostatic tissue.

"A water-based saw palmetto preparation, such as a tea, would give little or no benefit," says Tyler.

VITEX FOR FEMALE REPRODUCTIVE HEALTH

Actress Linda Lavin had hot flashes "that could take the chrome off a car." But when her doctor advised her to undergo hormone replacement therapy, she refused. "Menopause is a rite of passage," Lavin says. "It's not a disease." Lavin has joined the ranks of a growing number of women today who are seeking natural ways to deal with reproductive health issues. Whether they're plagued with painful periods or the symptoms associated with menopause, more women are turning to alternative therapies such as acupuncture, acupressure, aromatherapy, and herbal treatments. And when it comes to herbs, the treatment of choice for many women is vitex (Vitex agus castus)—also known as chasteberry—the fruit of a tree that women have relied on for centuries. "Many of the women I see in my practice use vitex to ease a number of symptoms associated with reproductive health," says Arnold Fox, M.D., a physician in Beverly Hills, California, who incorporates alternative therapies in his practice. "Most of them say that chasteberry helps them a great deal."

From premenstrual syndrome to menopause, reproductive health issues challenge women for most of their lives. But in the last 50 years, conventional medicine has often viewed such natural female processes as diseases. As a result, some doctors have advised women to undergo risky surgeries such as hysterectomy (removal of the uterus) and oophorectomy (removal of one or both ovaries) or to take synthetic hormones, which may relieve reproductive symptoms but may increase the risk of certain cancers and cause unpleasant side effects.

Before the advent of modern medicine, women turned to medicinal plants such as vitex to ease menstrual cramping, blunt the pain of childbirth, and alleviate uncomfortable symptoms that may accompany the onset of menopause. It is ironic that in an era marked by undreamed-of technological advances in medicine, more women are looking to those simpler times when nature provided remedies.

Take a look in your local health-food store or pharmacy. You're likely to find a number of natural medicines that wouldn't have been there ten years ago. But are such products safe to take? Vitex, by all accounts, is safe for moderate consumption. And many women report that it is capable of relieving the myriad, often painful, symptoms that signal changes within a woman's reproductive system.

The Menstrual Cycle

Menstruation is a normal part of a woman's reproductive cycle. The process begins when a girl enters puberty and continues until midlife, when menopause brings an end to her periods. Each month, when a woman's ovary releases an egg, it also secretes the hormones estrogen and progesterone. These hormones stimulate the endometrium (the tissue lining the uterus), encouraging it to thicken and engorge with blood so that it can nourish a fertilized egg. If the egg is not fertilized by a sperm, the ovary stops production of the hormones, which prompts the uterus to shed its lining and eliminate it in the menstrual flow. This process is repeated approximately every 28 days.

There are, however, problems or discomforts related to the reproductive process that can arise. Some of the more common problems, along with their conventional medical treatments, are discussed in the following sections.

Premenstrual Syndrome (PMS)

Menstruation can produce some discomfort, but the degree of severity differs from one woman to another. In the 10 to 14 days leading up to their periods, some women develop premenstrual syndrome (PMS), with symptoms such as irritability, anxiety, depression, mood swings, bloating, headaches, breast tenderness, fatigue, sugar craving, and weight gain.

"Sixty percent of women have enough symptoms due to PMS to suffer," says Christine Northrup, M.D., past president of the American Holistic Medical Association.

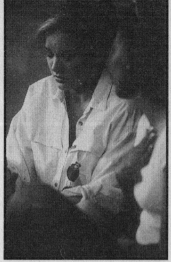
PMS may cause mood swings, anxiety, and irritability.

It used to be that many doctors considered such symptoms to be psychological, if they conceded that they existed at all. Now we know that PMS is a physical condition that may cause extreme discomfort in many women.

But we don't know for certain what causes PMS. Hormonal, nutritional, and psychological factors are all possibilities. In and of themselves, the symptoms of PMS are not indicative of disease. But if your period brings severe pain and discomfort, you should discuss it with your doctor, who can check for an underlying cause, such as endometriosis (the growth of endometrial tissue outside of the uterus, such as on the intestines) or the presence of an ovarian cyst (a fluid-filled sac that forms in an ovary).

Amenorrhea (Lack of Bleeding)

Amenorrhea is characterized by lack of menstruation. Any number of factors may prevent you from having your monthly period. If you are pregnant, for example, you won't menstruate until well after the baby is born. Amenorrhea also may result from delayed onset of puberty, excessive exercise, an increase in psy-

Vitex at a Glance

Latin name: *Vitex agnus castus*

Description: Vitex has also been called chasteberry, monk's pepper, cloister pepper, Indian spice, sage tree, hemp tree, and wild pepper. Vitex is an aromatic shrub or small tree that produces lavender-colored flowers and a fruit with an odor that is peppery and aromatic. The odor is apparent because vitex contains a number of volatile oils.

chological stress, illness, or anorexia nervosa, a condition marked by refusal to eat and extreme weight loss.

An imbalance in your hormone levels may also disrupt your menstrual cycle and cause missed periods. In the short term, such an imbalance is not usually serious. However, if you are not having periods, you may not be producing enough progesterone; a long-term lack of progesterone increases your risk of developing uterine diseases, such as endometrial cancer.

Depending on the cause of your lack of periods, you may be able to take steps to reestablish normal menstruation. If your lifestyle is the suspected cause of your amenorrhea, you might need to find ways to lessen the stress in your life or reduce an overzealous exercise regime. For

Habitat: Vitex is native to southern Europe and the Middle East but has become naturalized in most warm regions. The small tree grows best in sandy, or loamy, well-drained soil in full sun.

disorders such as anorexia or endometriosis, medical treatment of the condition may also result in a return of periods. If your failure to menstruate is caused by a hormonal irregularity, a holistic practitioner might suggest diet and lifestyle changes, herbs, acupuncture, and other natural treatments. A conventional doctor, on the other hand, might suggest that you undergo treatment to replace the missing hormones. In rare cases, surgery is necessary to remove a benign or malignant growth that is affecting the menstrual cycle.

Dysmenorrhea (Painful Periods)

If your period is painful and marked by excessive clotting, you may have dysmenorrhea. For some women, dysmenorrhea is typical for them.

Vitex Through History

Vitex got its most common folk name because the herb was once used to keep people chaste. From ancient times, vitex has been used to reduce sexual desire, especially in men.

During the Middle Ages, vitex was often added to meals at monasteries, where it got the nicknames monk's pepper and cloister pepper.

In rare cases, however, it may be caused by endometriosis, fibroids (noncancerous tumors), or other abnormal growths in the uterus.

Painful periods also may be caused by hormonal changes during your menstrual cycle. Your body could be making an excess of prostaglandins, hormone-like chemicals that cause uterine contractions during menstruation and labor. Contractions during menstruation ensure that all menstrual blood and unwanted tissue are expelled from your body. But excess prostaglandins may cause repeated contractions, and even spasms, which you may experience as painful cramping.

If your periods are mildly painful, you may find that herbs such as valerian, hop, cramp bark, chamomile, and black haw bark, or over-the counter analgesics such as aspirin or aceta-

Vitex has always been an important remedy in Europe for controlling and regulating the female reproductive system. Women have used vitex to treat irregular periods and other menstrual problems, including amenorrhea and dysmenorrhea, and to help promote fertility.

In addition, midwives gave patients vitex to ease the pains associated with childbirth. Later, when women entered menopause, they also took the herb to help them through the transition.

minophen help. You can also try ibuprofen, mefanamic acid, or naproxen, which inhibit the synthesis of prostaglandins. In more severe cases, you might want to visit a naturopathic physician or licensed acupuncturist for a treatment plan or see a conventional physician, who may prescribe birth control pills or progesterone, which may alter your hormone levels and relieve your pain.

Menorrhagia
(Heavy Menstrual Flow)

Menorrhagia is marked by heavy menstrual flow. The condition may result from stress, a hormonal imbalance, endometriosis, pelvic lesions or infections, or uterine growths such as fibroids. You may suspect menorrhagia if your periods last longer than eight days, your tampons or napkins are saturated with large blood clots, or you have to change your tampon or pad more than every one to two hours.

Usually menorrhagia is not a problem. But excessive bleeding may signal other more serious problems, including lack of ovulation, low levels of progesterone or other hormonal imbalance, an excess of certain prostaglandins, uterine fibroids, pelvic infection, or endometriosis. Untreated, menorrhagia may lead to iron-deficiency anemia.

If your periods are excessively heavy, your doctor may suggest that you take iron and folic acid supplements to treat or prevent anemia. Your doctor may also prescribe an antiprostaglandin analgesic such as ibuprofen or naproxen for pain and hormones such as progesterone and birth control pills to override imbalances.

You also may experience relief from a minor surgical procedure called dilation and curettage (D & C). Although D & C is basically a diagnostic procedure, it sometimes also relieves excessive menstrual flow either temporarily or permanently. In a D & C, the doctor widens the cervical opening, then uses a scraping instrument or gentle suction to remove the inner layers of the uterus. If this procedure itself does not provide relief, it may help the doctor to identify the underlying cause of the excessive bleeding so that it can be treated.

Menopause

The end of menstruation may bring about as many symptoms as the process itself. Menopause is a term doctors use to describe the months or years immediately before and after a woman experiences her final menstrual period.

Menopause is part of a woman's natural life cycle. In mid-life, usually during her 40s, a woman's ovaries begin to slow their release of eggs. Eventually, they stop releasing eggs, and the woman can no longer bear children. (In a healthy woman, this generally occurs between the ages of 45 and 55.) At the same time, production of estrogen and progesterone decreases significantly. Due to these changes, a woman may experience a variety of symptoms, including hot flashes, fatigue, and vaginal dryness.

In early human history, few women lived beyond menopause. Today, the average life expectancy for women is 79. That means that many of the 43 million women in America undergoing menopause at any given time will live a third of their lives after their childbearing years have ended. To ensure the quality of those years, it's important for women to continue to maintain good reproductive health.

Not every woman experiences problems with menopause. Nineteen percent of respondents reported that they never experienced hot flashes, according to a recent Massachusetts Women's Health Study of more than 8,000 women ages 45 to 55. The study also found that:

• On average, women stop having menstrual periods at age 51. Some women enter menopause as early as age 40, and a small percentage of women don't experience menopause until they reach age 60.

- Smokers enter menopause one to two years earlier than nonsmokers and ex-smokers.

- For most women, menopause lasts about four years.

Nature has a way of letting you know when you're about to stop having your monthly periods. A few years beforehand, you may notice that you're beginning to have irregular periods or that you're producing a lighter-than-usual menstrual flow. You may also begin to experience

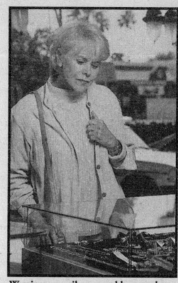

Wearing an easily removable outer layer of clothing can help you cool off quickly when a hot flash strikes.

symptoms such as hot flashes and mood swings. Such symptoms usually disappear as your body adjusts to the changes it's undergoing.

But menopause may cause more serious problems, too. The estrogen produced by the ovaries during the childbearing years also helps your bones to hold onto calcium. As your body produces less estrogen, your bones have trouble absorbing calcium, which increases your risk of developing osteoporosis (a thinning of the bones that makes them more fragile and prone to breakage). The decrease in estrogen may also contribute to a rise in your blood cholesterol levels, leaving you at greater risk for developing a heart attack or stroke.

As a response to these risks, as well as to the discomforts of menopause, hormone replacement therapy has become the first line of treatment. Each year, about 30 percent of American women ages 40 to 60 undergo the treatment.

Estrogen replacement therapy came into vogue in 1966 with the publication of a book by Robert A. Wilson, M.D., called *Feminine Forever.* Wilson expounded the view that menopause is a disease caused by a deficiency of estrogen. Without the hormone, Wilson maintained, women become sexless "caricatures of their former selves...the equivalent of a eunuch." By replacing lost estrogen, Wilson proposed, women could remain "feminine forever."

But subsequent research on hormone replacement in menopausal women has been flawed and contradictory, says Sandra Coney, author of *The Menopause Industry: How the Medical Establishment Exploits Women.*

"Women on estrogen require more doctor visits; they require regular mammograms; they need more tests; and they're more likely to end up having endometrial biopsies and hysterectomies," Coney argues.

A decade after publication of Wilson's book, in fact, researchers discovered a firm link between estrogen replacement and development of uterine cancer. To reduce that risk, drug makers began adding synthetic progesterone to supplement the estrogen and combat that risk.

In addition, while women once were put on hormone therapy for only several months to a year, many now are being advised to continue taking hormones for the rest of their lives.

The reason some doctors recommend long-term hormone replacement is that they believe the treatment may prevent their patients from having heart attacks, which are far more prevalent among postmenopausal women than among premenopausal women. Adding estrogen to a woman's body also appears to increase HDL, or beneficial, cholesterol, and lower LDL, the damage-causing form of cholesterol. In addition, estrogen replacement therapy increases blood flow to the heart by prompting arteries to expand, thus lowering a woman's chances of developing abnormal blood clots that may lead to heart attacks.

The side effects of estrogen therapy, however, include increased risk of some types of cancer, gallstones, strokes, nausea, PMS-like symptoms, breast tenderness, depression, liver disorders, enlargement of uterine fibroids, fluid retention, blood sugar disturbances, and headaches. And estrogen therapy alone increases the risk of endometrial cancer.

To reduce the risk of endometrial cancer, you can take estrogen with progesterone. Some more-holistically oriented physicians recommend micronized progesterone, a natural form of the hormone made from yams. Depending on how it is administered, however, adding progesterone to estrogen replacement therapy can cause monthly periods.

Hormone replacement therapy—administered in supplements or a skin patch—also has been

Prescription for Vitex

Capsules: 1 to 2 capsules per day

Tincture: ¼ to ½ teaspoon one to two times per day

recommended to help prevent osteoporosis, particularly if there is a family history of the condition. And your doctor also may prescribe vaginal estrogen cream to stop the thinning of vaginal tissues and to improve lubrication.

You should not take hormone replacement therapy if you have had breast cancer, endometrial cancer, or liver disease, because it might cause a recurrence of those problems.

Using Vitex

Although women have been using vitex for centuries, scientists still do not know exactly how vitex's healing effects occur. We know that vitex's constituents include monoterpenes, such as agnuside, eurostoside, and aucubin, as well as the flavonoids casticin, penduletin, and their derivatives. It is likely that vitex's beneficial effects

---

Menopause Tea
Vitex: 2 parts
St. John's wort: 1 part
Motherwort: 2 parts
Black cohosh root: 1 part

Steep 2 teaspoons of the herb mixture per cup of boiling water for 15 minutes. Drink about three cups a day. If combining these herbs in tincture form, take ½ to 1 teaspoon two to three times a day.

---

are related to the combination of its constituents.

What preliminary research does indicate is that vitex appears to correct a relative deficiency of progesterone, although none of the known constituents of vitex appears to have hormonal activity. Vitex appears to correct the progesterone deficiency indirectly, by affecting the hormone production of the pituitary gland. German tests of laboratory animals, for example, have revealed that vitex stimulates release of luteinizing hormone (LH), which prepares the body for pregnancy, and inhibits the release of follicle-stimulating hormone (FSH), which is normally released in the first half of the menstrual cycle to prepare for ovulation and the "ripening" of the egg.

Herbal healers long have used vitex—either alone or in combination with herbs such as black cohosh (Cimicifuga racemosa)—to treat

---

Is Vitex Safe?

Used moderately, in prescribed doses, vitex appears to be safe. There have been no reports of the herb causing toxic reactions in animals or humans. However, it is wise to consult a holistically oriented physician before trying vitex.

amenorrhea, dysmenorrhea, PMS, endometriosis, and menopause. And clinical studies appear to corroborate the use of such folk remedies. At a clinic in London, Dr. Alan Stewart gave 30 women with premenstrual symptoms 1.5 grams a day of dried vitex in capsule form. Stewart found that the women reported a 60 percent reduction in symptoms such as anxiety, nervous tension, insomnia, and mood changes.

Vitex also has been used effectively to treat many of the symptoms associated with menopause. Sometimes the herb is used alone, and sometimes it is combined with other herbs that nourish the female glandular system. These include angelica (*Angelica sinensis,* or dong quai), licorice root *(Glycyrrhiza glabra),* and black cohosh.

Also effective have been combinations of vitex, motherwort *(Leonurus cardiaca),* and wild yam *(Dioscorea villosa),* which help to calm the rapid heartbeat that often accompanies hot flashes.

If you suffer from painful periods or menopausal symptoms, it's important that you discuss the problem with your physician to rule out more serious causes. Then look into the pros and cons of taking conventional medicines. And don't overlook using vitex. By itself, or as a supplement to pharmaceuticals, vitex may provide the relief you're seeking.

FEVERFEW FOR MIGRAINES

*It begins like a wisp of smoke, curling around her head. And then the space between her eyebrows seems to explode in pain that lasts for days at a time. "It's the worst pain you can imagine," says Shannon, who lives in Miami, Florida, and has suffered for years from migraine headaches. "I've tried nearly everything, and nothing seems to help." Shannon may be a prime candidate for therapy using an herb called feverfew (*Tanacetum parthenium*). Once used to treat a variety of conditions, including headaches and fever, feverfew has recently been "rediscovered" by migraine sufferers, who are using the herb to blunt the sometimes crippling pain that accompanies their sudden and ill-understood attacks.*

For many of us, headaches top the list of common complaints. And migraines are by far the most painful and debilitating type of headache.

An intense migraine attack can floor victims, plaguing them with nausea and vertigo (dizziness) and confining them to bed. Although over-the-counter analgesics such as aspirin and ibuprofen work well to stop many types of headache pain, they're relatively ineffective when it comes to migraines. Prescription drugs don't work well for many migraine sufferers, and most have the potential for causing unwanted side effects. For those people, feverfew, an herb used centuries ago for its pain-killing properties, may hold the key. Scientists now know that feverfew contains chemicals that may prevent migraines. And the best news is that feverfew has few side effects. But is feverfew powerful enough to consistently take on the pain of migraines? "Feverfew works in about 50 percent of cases, which is not bad," says Arnold Fox, M.D., a physician in Beverly Hills, California, who prescribes the herb to many of his migraine patients. "I suggest that they give feverfew a try, along with stress-reduction techniques, which can be very effective."

Why Your Head Hurts

Doctors separate headaches into two categories: those that are caused by muscle contractions, and attacks brought on by vascular irregularities, such as expansion or contraction of blood vessels.

If your headache begins in the back of your neck and expands outward with a dull pain, you probably have a tension headache. Ninety percent of all headaches are thought to fall into this category. Tension headaches may be brought on by muscle contractions caused by poor posture, spinal misalignment, digestive problems, poor diet, or most often, stress.

Vascular problems account for so-called cluster headaches. Cluster headaches are extremely painful. They are often concentrated around the eye and may produce tears, facial flushing, and nasal congestion. Men seem to get them more often than women do.

But women are more likely to experience migraines. Indeed, migraines strike three times as many women as men.

Migraines can be debilitating. If you've ever had one, you may have been all but incapacitated by the pain and nausea that frequently accompany attacks. And just about anything may precipitate an attack: excessive caffeine, various foods or scents, dry winds, changes in altitude or seasons, hormonal fluctuations, taking birth control pills, missing a meal, or being in a stuffy room. Intense emotions, such as excitement or anger, also have brought on migraine attacks in some people. Even exercising, having sex, or eating very cold foods could lead to an episode.

In about 10 to 20 percent of migraine sufferers, the pain may be preceded by a visual warning. Such people may see a sort of "aura" that may include flickering points of light, blind spots, or zig-zagging lines. Rarely, migraine sufferers may also smell peculiar odors or notice that their limbs have become numb just prior to an attack.

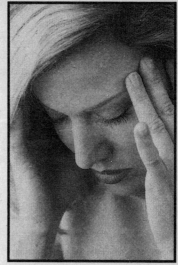

Migraines strike three times as many women as men.

(It's partly for this reason that some researchers think migraines are nerve-related, or neurological, in origin.) Most people who get migraines, however, are knocked for a loop with no warning at all.

A migraine headache usually starts with an intense, throbbing pain on one side of the head. Usually the pain begins to spread. And often, victims experience nausea and vomiting as well. Oversensitivity to stimuli is also a symptom of migraines. You may be especially aware of lights, odors, and sounds. This phenomenon probably occurs because blood vessels in your brain are overreacting by contracting and expanding abnormally.

Symptoms vary from person to person and may range in severity. A migraine headache may last a few hours, or it could make your life miserable for up to three days. Why you get migraines, however, is not clearly understood.

Researchers have linked migraine symptoms to changes in the diameter of blood vessels in the head. At first, the vessels constrict. Then, as the pain begins, they dilate. What scientists don't know is why these changes occur.

One theory is that they result from an imbalance in a mood-regulating brain chemical called sero-

Feverfew at a Glance

Latin names: *Tanacetum parthenium; Chrysanthemum parthenium*

Description: Feverfew is a hardy plant that may prosper as a biennial or perennial, depending on climate and soil conditions. The herb produces a branched, tufted root and finely furrowed stems with several branches. Feverfew's flowers look somewhat like those of some varieties of chamomile. It has a round, central yellow floret surrounded by white

tonin. Hormones probably also play a role in the development of migraine headaches. There seems to be a strong connection between estrogen levels and migraines. That may explain why more women than men experience migraines and why attacks often seem to occur just before, during, or after a woman's menstrual period. Migraine headaches, moreover, seem to run in families, spurring some researchers to speculate that victims have a "migraine gene" that predisposes them to attacks.

Conventional Drugs

There are several over-the-counter and prescription medicines that may shorten the duration and lessen the intensity of a migraine

---

petals. Feverfew produces finely cut green leaves, unlike the more feathery leaves of chamomile. Feverfew's leaves are strongly scented and have a bitter taste. The plant may grow to two or three feet tall (unlike the smaller chamomile, which rarely grows larger than a foot tall). It flowers midsummer through fall.

Habitat: Feverfew is native to central and southern Europe and has become naturalized in many temperate parts of the world, including areas of North America.

attack. Finding the right drug or combination of drugs may take some trial and error.

For people who experience migraines infrequently and whose migraines don't totally knock them off their feet, an over-the-counter analgesic, such as aspirin, ibuprofen, acetaminophen, or naproxen sodium, may help to ease migraine pain. Sometimes, these are more effective when combined with caffeine and taken early in the attack.

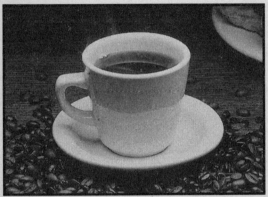

Caffeine may help ease migraine pain.

To help combat other symptoms of migraines, a doctor may have you try specific medications. For example, your doctor may prescribe the drug metoclopramide (Clopra, Octamide, Reclomide, Reglan). Taken at the first sign of a migraine attack, the drug helps to reduce nausea. Metoclopramide, however, may cause mild to severe depression in some people. Therefore, you need to inform your doctor if you have ever suffered from depression. Other common side effects of metoclopramide include drowsiness, fatigue, listlessness, or restlessness.

Some people find that prescription analgesics such as aspirin or acetaminophen combined with codeine or another narcotic are effective in alleviating migraine pain. But such drugs may be habit-forming (meaning they may cause mental or physical dependence) and, for some patients, may increase nausea and vomiting. And if the drug is stopped suddenly, the patient may experience withdrawal symptoms.

Narcotics such as codeine may also block the action of other medications, including prophylactic drugs that your doctor might prescribe to prevent you from having migraine attacks. And if you develop a dependence on caffeine and codeine, you could blunt the effectiveness of your body's natural pain killers, chemicals known as endorphins.

For severe migraine attacks, your doctor may prescribe a drug called sumatriptan (Imitrex), which has brought dramatic relief to some migraine sufferers. It will not reduce the number of migraines you experience, but it may help treat an acute attack. It is available as an injection (which works most rapidly), a nasal spray, or a pill (which takes longest to ease pain).

Sumatriptan, however, can cause serious side effects. Although rare, serious heart conditions have developed in some people who had existing cardiac problems and took the drug. More common side effects include a burning sensation, dizziness or vertigo, a feeling of heaviness or tightness, mouth and tongue discomfort, muscle weakness, neck pain and stiffness, numbness, and sore throat.

Another option for severe migraine attacks is medication containing ergotamine or dihydroergotamine. These medications act quickly to constrict blood vessels and reduce painful

Feverfew Through History

Most herbal historians have assumed that feverfew's name derives from the Latin *febrifugia*, which means "driver out of fevers." Roman physicians used it widely for just that purpose.

But modern herbalist Michael Castleman says that feverfew's name is a misnomer. "Ancient physicians, including Dioscorides and Galen, used its Greek name, *parthenion*," Castleman says, "and they prescribed the herb for menstrual and birth-related problems—not fever."

During the Middle Ages, Castleman says, the herb was known as featherfoil because of its feathery, fernlike leaves. That name eventually corrupted into

inflammation caused by migraines. Some forms also contain medications to combat nausea and vomiting or to help the patient relax and sleep.

Ergotamine-containing products may also have serious side effects, which you should discuss with your physician. Excessive use of ergotamine, for example, may lead to ergot poisoning, producing symptoms including headaches, leg pain when walking, general muscle pain, numbness, a feeling of coldness, and abnormal paleness of the fingers and toes. Untreated, ergot poisoning could lead to gangrene, in which lack of blood supply causes tissues to die. Some er-

featherfew, and from there, it's not difficult to see how the name may have evolved into feverfew.

Because of that nickname, Castleman says, herbalists began prescribing it as a treatment for fevers. Peasants began to plant the herb around their homes in hopes of warding off pestilent fevers. And early North American settlers carried feverfew to these shores to treat malaria, a major killer in the New World. For centuries thereafter, feverfew use slid into the background, being prescribed by only those herbalists who appreciated its broader applications.

It's only been recently that this member of the chrysanthemum family has been "rediscovered" and "reapplied." Now, some scientists think that feverfew may hold the key to treating, not fevers, but migraine headaches.

gotamine medications may cause fluid retention, high blood pressure, and vertigo.

If your migraines are severe — if you experience three or more attacks a month — your doctor may want you to take a daily prophylactic medicine to prevent the episodes from occurring.

Verapamil (Calan, Isoptin, Verelan), a calcium-channel-blocking drug, has prevented migraines in some people. But the drug has the potential for causing congestive heart failure, constipation, dizziness, fatigue, fluid retention, low blood pressure, and nausea.

Growing Your Own

Feverfew makes a beautiful addition to any flower garden. Its soft, light-green serrated leaves form mounds that can grow as high as two feet. In summer and well into fall, these leaf mounds will sprout flowers that resemble daisies.

Feverfew is also easy to grow; it is an undemanding plant. It thrives in any type of well-drained soil and will even self-sow into crevices in walls and between paving stones.

Feverfew seeds are sold under several names. In some catalogs, you may find feverfew listed as *Matricaria eximia* (Feverfew's cousin, chamomile, is called *Matricaria recutita*). The herb also comes in several

Propranolol (Inderal), a medicine often prescribed to lower blood pressure, also may help prevent migraines. Propranolol is a beta-adrenergic blocker that works by preventing blood vessels from constricting. Although it is effective for some migraine sufferers, it may cause side effects in others. Side effects may include abdominal cramps, colitis (inflammation of the large intestine), congestive heart failure, constipation, decreased sexual ability, depression, diarrhea, breathing difficulties, disorientation, dry eyes, fever with sore throat, hair loss, hallucinations, headache, light-headedness, lupus erythematosus (a chronic inflammatory disease that

varieties. Some produce double flowers, yellow flowers, or golden foliage. Some of the compact double varieties make especially attractive container plants. *Aureum,* a type of feverfew, has golden leaves that remain bright even in winter.

Sow feverfew seeds in spring if you want your plants to bloom by midsummer. Once the plants are big enough, you may reproduce them by taking cuttings, although the process can be difficult with this type of herb. If you live in cool regions, you may divide plants in spring or fall.

In the far north, feverfew is a short-lived perennial, so try to maintain a good supply of new plants. That way you'll never be without a ready source of migraine medicine.

effects many systems of the body), nausea, rash, slow heartbeat, and fatigue.

Propranolol may also mask symptoms of low blood sugar, alter blood-sugar levels, and interact with other medications. If you use propranolol, don't suddenly stop taking it. Otherwise, you could experience chest pain or even have a heart attack. If you wish to stop taking the drug, ask your doctor to gradually decrease your dosage.

If you're one of those migraine sufferers who have had little success using pharmaceutical drugs, you may want to talk with your doctor about feverfew. "I would rather take feverfew for a migraine than take a prescription drug," says medical botanist James Duke, Ph.D., former chief of the U.S. Department of Agriculture's Medicinal Plant Laboratory. "Feverfew works just as effectively as pharmaceuticals, and it has no serious side effects, although it occasionally causes mouth ulcers in those who chew it, which is usually obviated [prevented] by taking the capsule."

Using Feverfew

Feverfew's flowers look similar to chamomile's, and indeed, both herbs belong to the chrysanthemum family. But unlike chamomile, feverfew is a shrub with large, cut-out leaves—more leaves than chamomile. Both herbs help to control spasms. Chamomile is used most often to treat digestive problems. And feverfew holds a hallowed spot in the annals of folk medicine as a remedy for headaches—especially stubborn ones.

"Feverfew is one of the best herbal remedies I know of for migraines," says Connie Grauds, an herbalist who founded the Association of Natural Medicine Pharmacists.

Many researchers would agree with Grauds, and with her forebear, English herbalist John Gerard, who declared in 1633 that feverfew is "very good for them that are giddie in the head." A century later, herbalist John Hill noted that "in the worst headache, this herb exceeds whatever else is known."

Feverfew contains compounds called parthenolides, which appear to help control expansion and contraction of blood vessels in the head. When you begin to get a migraine, your brain releases the neurotransmitter serotonin, and your blood vessels constrict. Feverfew appears to counteract your brain's order by causing blood vessels to dilate. Thus, feverfew enhances the "tone" of blood vessels, as does magnesium, which is also considered to be a helpful nutrient for controlling migraine headaches.

In addition, feverfew appears to neutralize chemicals called prostaglandins, some of which are linked to pain and inflammation. Because it stops production of inflammatory chemicals, feverfew also has a history as a treatment for arthritis.

But no one really knows why feverfew performs in these ways. In 1978, scientists speculated in the British medical journal *Lancet* that feverfew might share some properties with aspirin. Two years later, *Lancet* published a study that appeared to confirm this theory. Parthenolides, however, appear to block prostaglandin production earlier in the process than does aspirin.

Among feverfew's main constituents are substances known as sequiterpene lactones (parthenolides are among them). Like aspirin, these chemicals inhibit platelet aggregation (the clotting of blood cells). In several studies done in test tubes, feverfew extracts have slowed the formation of clotlike substances on collagen (fibrous tissue).

Is Feverfew Safe?

Used as directed, feverfew is safe. There have been no reports of feverfew causing uterine contractions, but the herb has a long folk history as a promoter of

And in 1985, scientists theorized in the *British Medical Journal* that feverfew may contain chemical substances that encourage smooth muscle cells to be less responsive to the body chemicals that trigger migraine muscle spasms.

A Bit of Feverfew History

While scientific research continues to expand our knowledge of how feverfew works, it was word of mouth that originally got scientists to notice the herb.

In the late 1970s, the wife of the chief medical officer of Great Britain's National Coal Board suffered greatly from migraine headaches. A local coal miner heard about the woman's problem and told her he had also been a long-time migraine sufferer until he started chewing a couple of feverfew leaves each day. How the miner originally heard about this folk remedy is a mystery, but the woman tried it anyway and noticed almost immediately that the frequency and

menstruation, so don't use it if you are pregnant. Feverfew also may cause sores inside the mouth, and some people have reported experiencing abdominal pains after ingesting it. Feverfew may inhibit blood clotting, so don't use it if you are on an anticoagulant (blood-thinning) medication.

severity of her headaches decreased. After taking feverfew for 14 months, her migraines stopped completely.

Impressed by his wife's recovery, her husband relayed the story to Dr. E. Stewart Johnson of the City of London Migraine Clinic. Johnson was intrigued and decided to test feverfew on his patients. He started out by administering feverfew leaves to ten migraine sufferers at the clinic. At the end of the trial, three of the patients reported that their headaches had been cured. The other seven noted significant improvement in their symptoms.

Johnson then decided to test feverfew on a grander scale. He gave the herb to 270 migraine patients who had had little success from using conventional medicines. Johnson separated the patients into two groups. One group was given feverfew; the other received a placebo (dummy pill). The results of the test were dramatic. Seventy percent of the patients who took feverfew said they believed that the herb had diminished the intensity and frequency of their attacks. Most of the people in the placebo group continued to suffer from migraines.

Lancet later published the results of a rigorous clinical trial in which researchers gave 72 migraine patients either a dummy pill or a capsule a day of powdered freeze-dried feverfew (each capsule contained the equivalent of two medium-size feverfew leaves). None of the patients in the study knew whether they were taking the dummy pill or the feverfew pill. The researchers discovered that feverfew eliminated migraine headaches in 24 percent of the patients who took the herb, and the rest of the subjects in the feverfew group experienced much milder migraine attacks. Patients who were taking the dummy pill, however, suffered a variety of migraine symptoms during the six months of the study; those side effects included headaches, nausea, and vomiting. The symptoms were so severe that two of the subjects who were taking the dummy pills guessed that they were taking the useless medicine, left the study, and demanded to take feverfew. Once they did, their headaches stopped.

Can Feverfew Help You?

If you suffer from migraine headaches, don't throw away your prescription medicines. They may prove to be invaluable to you if you suffer a severe migraine attack. But if feverfew's clinical track record impresses you, you may want to talk to a holistically oriented physician about taking the herb to prevent your headaches from occurring. That seems to be how feverfew works best.

"Feverfew has no beneficial effect on migraine attacks once they're in gear," according to pharmacognosist Varro E. Tyler, Ph.D, professor emeritus at the Purdue University School of Pharmacy in Indiana. "It works as a preventive, and that means taking it regularly over a long period."

Other herbalists, however, maintain that feverfew can help to lessen the intensity of migraine attacks that have already begun. You and your doctor will have to experiment with the herb to determine how it works best for you and how you should take it.

Prescription for Feverfew

Capsules: Take a pill or capsule containing 85 milligrams of the leaf every day. In clinical trials, the parthenolide content of feverfew has ranged from 0.4 percent to 0.6 percent, and a quantity of the herb containing 250 micrograms of parthenolide is considered to be an adequate daily dose to prevent migraines. To offset a migraine attack that has just begun, take three or four feverfew capsules or leaves immediately and continue every four hours. Do not exceed 12 capsules in a day.

Leaves: A report in the journal *Lancet* shows that some pills and capsules contain only trace amounts of

You can buy feverfew as a tea or in tablet or tincture form, probably at your local drugstore or health-food store. But many herbalists say that feverfew works best if it is taken when fresh. Feverfew isn't difficult to grow, so you may want to consider adding it to your back-yard garden or cultivating it in a pot on your patio.

Then just harvest a few of the leaves every day and add them to salads or sandwiches. If migraines have been keeping you down, you may just find that feverfew makes the best lunch you'll ever eat.

---

the herb. And some studies indicate that best results are obtained from consuming the whole leaf. Indeed, the main study that did not show beneficial effects of feverfew on migraines used standardized capsules of alcohol-extracted powder rather than capsules containing the whole leaf. And test-tube studies show that whole-plant extracts are superior to isolated parthenolides. Thus, you may be better off growing your own feverfew and heading out to the garden every morning. You can pick enough leaves off the plant in the summer to tide you over until the following spring, when the plant comes back above ground and produces leaves again.

Tea: Steep 1 teaspoon feverfew leaves in 1 cup water for 10 minutes. Drink up to two cups a day.

CHROMIUM
FOR DIABETES

A little over a year ago, Janet's doctor told her she had developed a form of diabetes that most often strikes people in midlife. Fortunately, Janet would not have to take daily insulin injections. But she would have to control her blood sugar levels for the rest of her life. "My doctor wanted to put me on medication, but I told him that I wanted to try natural methods first," says Janet, a newspaper editor in Ohio. Janet embarked on a well-balanced diet and began walking two miles a day. She had also read that a natural supplement called chromium had helped some people to regulate their metabolism and sugar levels. Janet decided to give the supplement a try. Each day she took 500 milligrams of chromium. "When I started," she says, "I had a blood sugar reading of 160. After a couple of weeks, the chromium brought my level down to 87."

Since the 1950s, researchers have known that chromium plays a key role in the processes underlying one of the most serious diseases in our country—diabetes. Diabetes afflicts as many as 20 million people in the United States and can lead to serious complications, including blindness, gangrene (death of tissue, which usually requires amputation of the affected area), kidney disease, heart attacks, and strokes.

Doctors have at their disposal a variety of drugs that can help people with diabetes to keep blood sugar levels in check. But many of these medicines have undesirable side effects. As a result, more people like Janet are turning to natural alternatives, such as chromium, which many people say has helped them to control their diabetes. But is chromium safe, and does it really work?

What Is Diabetes?

Diabetes mellitus, the most common disorder of the endocrine system, is caused by disruptions in blood levels of insulin, a pancreatic hormone that helps your body to convert blood glucose, or sugar, into energy. One of the world's most insidious killers, diabetes comes in two major forms.

Type I diabetes, also known as insulin-dependent (IDDM) or juvenile-onset diabetes, occurs when the pancreas is unable to produce enough insulin. Because the body is therefore unable to use the glucose in the blood, it tries to produce energy by burning fat and muscle.

We're not entirely sure what causes this form of the disease, but it appears to be an autoimmune disorder in which the person's immune system attacks the pancreas. Genes may be involved: New research suggests that many people with Type I diabetes may have a genetic predisposition to the disease that is triggered by a viral infection.

Type I diabetes usually strikes people under the age of 30 and requires lifelong administration of daily insulin, so that the body can properly use glucose for energy. To regulate their insulin doses, people with Type I diabetes must take regular blood sugar readings.

Type II diabetes is closely linked to obesity.

Type II diabetes, also known as adult-onset or noninsulin-dependent diabetes (NIDDM), is most often diagnosed in people over the age of 40. About 90 percent of people with diabetes suffer from this form of the disease. People with Type II diabetes may have sufficient, or even excess, amounts of insulin, but their bodies become unable to use the hormone effectively.

There appears to be a strong link between Type II diabetes and obesity (defined as being more than 20 percent above desired body weight). Excessive food consumption boosts blood glucose levels, but the body loses its ability to properly convert the extra sugar into energy. It is this type of diabetes that generally responds well to diet and exercise adjustments and the use of chromium.

Why Worry About Diabetes?

Diabetes is dangerous because it can lead to so many potentially fatal illnesses. Researchers have found that both people with insulin-dependent Type I diabetes and people with noninsulin-dependent Type II diabetes have significantly lower-than-normal levels of protective antioxidants in their bodies. Thus, people with diabetes risk becoming disabled, or dying at an early age, from cardiovascular and other diseases.

In the long term, diabetes can damage your nervous system, kidneys, and cardiovascular and circulatory systems. In addition, diabetes reduces your resistance to infection. People with diabetes are also at increased risk of developing gum problems, urinary tract diseases, and mouth infections, such as thrush.

Diabetes is the leading cause of adult blindness in the United States. About ten years after diagnosis, half of all people with diabetes develop an eye disorder called diabetic retinopathy, which weakens the tiny blood vessels that supply blood to the retina and ultimately damages vision. People with diabetes are also more likely to develop cataracts and glaucoma.

Poor circulation leaves people with diabetes prone to skin ulcers, cramps, and gangrene, an infection that destroys tissue. And damaged blood vessels in the kidneys could lead to kidney failure.

A condition called diabetic neuropathy causes a gradual deterioration of the nervous system.

Chromium at a Glance

Description: Chromium is a trace mineral that your body needs to function.

Availability: Chromium is found in brewer's yeast, meats, chicken, shellfish (especially clams), corn oil, and whole grains.

The condition usually begins early in people with diabetes and affects the motor and sensory nerves. Among the consequences are slowed reflexes, loss of sensation, numbness, tingling in the legs, and impotence.

Fortunately, you can decrease your likelihood of developing many of the complications of diabetes by carefully regulating your blood sugar levels.

What Doctors Can Do

Diabetes cannot be cured, but it can be treated. If you have Type I diabetes, you must follow a plan developed especially for you by your doctor, diabetes educator, or other health-care provider.

If you have Type II diabetes, exercise and diet adjustments that help you shed excess weight

Action: Chromium plays a role in the regulation of the hormone insulin, which in turn regulates the way the body uses sugar.

Use: As an adjunct to diet and exercise, chromium supplementation may help people with Type II diabetes to maintain better control of blood sugar levels and perhaps reduce or eliminate the use of pharmaceutical medicines.

and keep it off may be enough to keep your disease under control. Your doctor may advise you to eat three small meals and three to four snacks a day so you maintain a proper balance between glucose and insulin in your blood. Your doctor is likely to refer you to a dietitian or diabetes educator who can help you plan meals and snacks.

You may also need to take an oral diabetes drug such as tolbutamide, glipizide, glyburide, chlorpropamide, metformin, acarbose, or troglitazone. However, these medications can cause side effects, including bloating, heartburn, nausea, and low blood sugar. Chlorpropamide may even lead to heart problems in some patients.

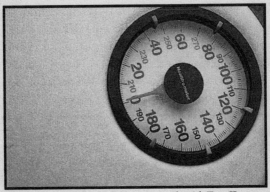

Losing excess weight can help some people with Type II diabetes avoid the need for medication.

One supplement that people with Type II diabetes may want to discuss with a physician experienced in holistic treatments is chromium. Chromium supplements appear to help many people with Type II diabetes. It may not only help lower blood glucose levels, it may improve glucose tolerance and help to hold down unhealthy forms of blood cholesterol.

What Is Chromium?

Chromium is a mineral that is essential for health. It is commonly found in brewer's yeast, meats, chicken, shellfish (especially clams), corn oil, and whole grains.

Chromium and a nutrient called nicotinic acid (a form of niacin) are essential components of the glucose tolerance factor (GTF), which regulates the actions of insulin in the human body. When you eat food, your blood glucose levels rise significantly. If your cells are resistant to insulin, they can't accept glucose. And if glucose can't get into your cells to produce energy, the blood sugar will be stored in your body as fat. Chromium appears able to combat cellular insulin resistance, enabling your cells to use the glucose you produce from food.

Some studies have found that chromium supplementation decreases fasting glucose levels and improves glucose tolerance in the body. Chromium appears to work even more effectively if combined with supplements of niacin, its partner in the GTF.

In 1980, scientists at Columbia University in New York reported in the *American Journal of Clinical Nutrition* that chromium helped elderly people with diabetes who took it in the form of brewer's yeast. "Chromium-rich brewer's yeast improved glucose tolerance and cholesterol in elderly normal and diabetic subjects," the researchers noted. "An improvement in insulin sensitivity also occurred with chromium supplementation."

In addition, Victoria J. K. Liu, Ph.D., at Indiana's Purdue University, found that people with high insulin levels are much more likely to have low chromium levels. People with Type II diabetes often have higher-than-normal insulin levels, but they are unable to use the insulin effectively. In some such people who have been given chromium, insulin and sugar levels went down.

"The abnormality," says Liu, "can be reversed in some cases with chromium supplementation."

Prescription for Chromium

To help bring blood sugar levels under control, take 200 to 300 micrograms of chromium with each meal; you may also wish to add a daily supplement of 100 milligrams of nicotinic acid. If you take insulin, this

It appears likely that the individuals who will benefit from chromium supplements are people with diabetes who are deficient in the mineral to begin with.

Scientists have not yet been able to establish a Recommended Daily Allowance for chromium. Some evidence indicates that an intake between 50 and 200 micrograms is safe and should be enough to prevent deficiency. But by some estimates, in the United States, the average chromium intake of men is 33 micrograms and of women, 25 micrograms.

Chromium levels, moreover, may be depleted in our bodies by strenuous exercise and physiological trauma, such as injuries, burns, and surgery. And as we grow older, our chromium supplies get lower and lower. Unfortunately, as we grow older, our bodies also become less capable of taking sugar from our blood to nourish our cells.

supplementation could reduce your need for the hormone. Some people with Type II diabetes find that one to three capsules (200 micrograms each) of chromium can significantly reduce blood sugar levels. Be sure to discuss your use of these supplements with a physician experienced in holistic as well as traditional medical treatments first.

Chromium may also be able to speed the healing of wounds, which often plague people with diabetes. Liu conducted a study to compare the healing time between rats fed a low-chromium diet and those fed a high-chromium diet. Fifteen days after undergoing major surgery, rats taking chromium exhibited a much more significant rate of healing than their low-chromium counterparts.

Not all studies of chromium have been conclusive, however. In some, chromium appeared to have little if any effect in improving glucose tolerance in people with diabetes. The results have been even more mixed when it comes to claims that chromium can help decrease body fat and increase lean (muscle) tissue.

Still, for many people, chromium has been a godsend in their attempts to control their blood sugar levels. Some, like Janet, have even been able to integrate the supplement with diet and

Is Chromium Safe?

There have been no adverse side effects reported in people who take chromium supplements. But, as with any substance you put in your body, exercise caution. Do not take more than 1,000 micrograms of chromium a day. If you plan on becoming pregnant,

exercise in order to avoid having to take pharmaceutical drugs.

If you have been diagnosed with Type II diabetes, discuss chromium supplements with a physician who has experience with holistic treatments as well as traditional diabetes treatments. In the meantime, do not discontinue any prescribed medication for diabetes. If you and your doctor decide that chromium is worth a try, you will have to be monitored, since your diet and medication may need to be adjusted.

Keep in mind that chromium is not a magic bullet by any means. You'll still have to implement major changes in your diet and activity level in order to control your diabetes. But chromium may help you in your fight to regain good health.

if you are pregnant, or if you are breast-feeding, consult your doctor before taking chromium or any other medicinal substance. Likewise, if you have diabetes, consult your doctor about the use of chromium before supplementing, and do not stop taking any prescribed diabetes medication without talking to your doctor first.

KAVA FOR ANXIETY

The year is 1768. English navigator Captain
James Cook has spent the last several months exploring
the uncharted islands of the South Seas. In a jungle
village on one such tropical isle, Cook is invited to
witness an ancient Polynesian ceremony. As drums beat
hypnotically, a group of girls ritually chews the root of a
sacred plant the islanders call kava kava. Following the
centuries-old practice of their grandmothers, the girls spit
the pulp into a bowl, and the mixture is stirred by the
village wise man. After asking the gods for their blessing,
the priest calls the village elders to partake of the brew.
Moments later, a serene expression transforms the
faces of the men. The kava spirit has spoken.

Today we know why Pacific island cultures so
revered the kava plant, which grows abun-
dantly throughout Polynesia. Kava contains
chemicals that seem to produce in many people
a profound sense of relaxation and well-being.
In Europe, a kava extract, marketed under the
brand name Kawain, has long been a popular
remedy for alleviating the tension and stress
that dog so many of us in the urban jungles of
the western world. Now kava is beginning to

make its mark in the United States. From Long Island to Los Angeles, kava can be found in health-food stores and on the shelves of conventional pharmacies. That's not surprising since modern science has begun to uncover indisputable links between stress and life-threatening illnesses, including cancer. But alleviating anxiety in a culture known for its angst is easier said than done. Benzodiazepines and other pharmaceuticals work effectively to reduce short-term tension. But taken on a regular basis, such medications may cause serious side effects, including addiction. Tranquilizers, moreover, may be lethal if washed down with alcohol. Kava's proponents—and the number is growing—say the herb is naturally safe to consume in moderate doses. But can kava stand up to the symptoms produced by the often stressful lifestyles so many of us lead today? Medical botanist James Duke, Ph.D., thinks so. "I predict we're going to see a boom in the sale of this herb," says Duke, former chief of the U.S. Department of Agriculture's Medicinal Plant Laboratory. "It's going to be similar to the boom we've seen with St. John's wort for depression."

What Is Anxiety?

Our bodies are designed to function in a wide variety of situations. We're even equipped with a warning system that kicks in when danger is present. In the days when our ancestors roamed the wild, danger lurked behind every tree. Humans hunted to live and were themselves hunted by predators. Under such circumstances, stress was a valuable ally. We needed stress to keep us on our toes—and keep us alive.

Today, we need no longer fear larger animals or enemies with war clubs skulking around every bush. Nonetheless, our biological warning system continues to sound the alarm if our brains think we're in danger. The siren is anxiety.

Anxiety results from the release of the chemical adrenaline into the bloodstream. This causes the heart rate to increase and breathing to become shallow and rapid. The liver releases energy-stimulating sugars, and muscles tense as the body prepares for "fight or flight."

Symptoms of Anxiety

Anxiety, an increasingly common ailment in our fast-paced society, produces a number of symptoms that may range from mild to alarming. Some of the most common symptoms include:

- Heart palpitations
- Sense of impending doom
- Inability to concentrate

The problem for many of us is that our warning systems are consistently going off, even though there's no real physical threat to our lives. Instead, we're perceiving danger when work piles up, the car conks out, or the kids are yelling.

Every time such modern stressors spur our alarm systems to kick in, our organs risk damage from the release of those powerful chemicals. Unless we do something to temper our reactions to stress, we may eventually acquire stress-related illnesses, such as headaches or high blood pressure. Or we could develop emotional anxiety disorders that can be just as crippling.

Anxiety Disorders

Anxiety disorders are widespread in our high-voltage culture. And they come in a staggering

---

- Muscle tension or aches
- Diarrhea or constipation
- Chest pain
- Dry mouth
- Excessive sweating
- Under- or overeating
- Insomnia
- Irritability
- Hyperventilation
- Loss of sex drive

---

variety. Phobias, for example, are irrational fears that nevertheless produce actual responses in our bodies. Perhaps you're afraid of flying, even though statistics indicate that flying is one of the safest forms of travel. Despite that knowledge, your muscles may tense and you may break out in a cold sweat when you even think about boarding an airplane.

One of the most severe and potentially debilitating phobias is agoraphobia, the fear of open spaces. Sometimes, for reasons that are not always clear, people become afraid to leave their homes. There have been accounts of such fear-ridden people who have literally spent years behind locked doors. Many who have recovered from agoraphobia say they became recluses because they feared having panic attacks.

Panic attacks are characterized by a sudden onset of extreme fear or tension. If you've ever

---

Kava at a Glance

Latin name: *Piper methysticum*

Description: Kava is a shrub that can grow to be several feet high. It produces heart-shaped leaves and short spikes rising from the base of leaf stems that may be densely covered with flowers. The rhizomes

had a panic attack, you may have thought at first that you were having a heart attack. One of

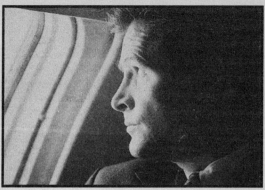

Fear of flying is a type of anxiety disorder called a phobia.

the symptoms of a panic attack is rapid heart-beat and shallow breathing. Remember the "fight or flight" response our ancient human underwent in the presence of danger? The same thing happens during a panic attack. Chemicals are released, and symptoms of profound anxiety overtake the body.

and roots of the kava plant are used medicinally. The root has a faint but characteristic odor and produces a bitter, pungent taste, which results in a slight local anesthetic (numb) feeling on the tongue.

Habitat: Kava is native to the Polynesian Islands but is cultivated widely and sold in most major cities. In Hawaii, more than 15 varieties are grown.

No one really knows why panic attacks occur. They seem to run in families, so there may be a genetic component. Studies of identical twins, for example, show that if one twin suffers from anxiety, the other is likely to be anxious as well.

Panic attacks may also result from long-term suppression of anxiety, as some psychiatrists theorize. Perhaps you grew up in a dysfunctional family. You may have pushed down the anxiety you felt at the time. Then, years later, the anxiety erupts when you least expect it.

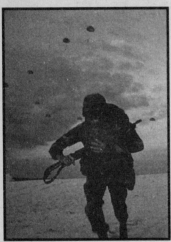

Sometimes such repressed anxiety takes the form of post-traumatic stress disorder. This condition made headlines in the years following the Vietnam War, after battle-scarred veterans began to demonstrate

Post-traumatic stress disorder can affect anyone who has gone through a horrific event.

bizarre, disturbing, or violent behavior during "flashbacks" to the horrors they experienced in the trenches and jungles of Southeast Asia. Thirty years ago, post-traumatic stress disorder was misunderstood by most people. Today we know that anyone who has undergone a horrific event — a catastrophic accident, child abuse, or rape, for example — may later develop anxiety-related problems with serious consequences.

Another illness caused by anxiety is known as obsessive-compulsive disorder. People with obsessive-compulsive disorder feel compelled to act out their irrational thoughts. They may, for example, feel an overwhelming need to check over and over again that they turned off the coffee pot or locked the door at bedtime. In severe cases, people with the disorder may spend hours indulging in repetitive behaviors, such as washing their hands or cleaning their homes.

Free-floating, or general, anxiety is perhaps the most common stress-related malady in our culture. Free-floating anxiety is a reaction to the stress we all feel from living in an increasingly complex world. Sometimes we may feel anxious for no apparent reason. Or we may feel a sense of impending doom as we "wait for the ax to fall" or for "the other shoe to drop." Generalized anxiety afflicts twice as many women as men and is more common among adults than children. It's also quite difficult to treat, because it has no readily identifiable source.

Of course, it's perfectly normal to feel anxious if we are facing a difficult situation. Changing jobs, moving to another town, or being separated from a loved one is sure to produce a certain level of stress in most people. Usually, symptoms caused by stressful incidents are temporary and disappear after we've dealt with the change or conflict in our lives.

But when symptoms of anxiety remain long after problems have been solved, or when we feel anxious and can't figure out why, we have a condition that needs treatment. Anxiety disorders may be mild, occurring periodically as we face life's challenges, or the symptoms may be incapacitating, requiring hospitalization. Usually they lie somewhere in the middle of the spectrum.

In addition to buried trauma, genetic predisposition, and sociological stress factors, anxiety may be caused by reactions to medications or by allergies. Food sensitivities may precipitate feelings of anxiety. Or you may experience symptoms after suddenly stopping regular use of drugs such as nicotine, alcohol, or caffeine.

If you are suffering from anxiety, it is important that you first rule out possible physical causes. Some illnesses, such as hyperthyroidism, may produce symptoms that resemble those of anxiety. In addition, certain heart disorders may cause rapid heartbeat, a symptom often associated with anxiety.

If you and your doctor determine that your symptoms are a reaction to stress, there are a number of conventional drugs and psychotherapeutic approaches that may help you.

Seeing a Therapist

Your first line of treatment may be psychotherapy, in which you and a qualified therapist attempt to identify the emotional conflicts that may form the basis of your anxiety. Psychotherapy is a term comprising many techniques.

Behavior modification therapy focuses on changing the patterns of behavior that may be causing you to feel anxious. If you're afraid to fly, for example, behavior modification therapy could teach you how to approach your fear rationally and eventually conquer it.

Cognitive therapy, on the other hand, concentrates on changing the way you think about an anxiety-provoking stressor. Sometimes simply changing your perception of a situation from negative to positive is enough to reduce your symptoms of anxiety.

Psychotherapy may be goal oriented, ending after you have achieved desired results. Or therapy may go on for months or years as you attempt to better understand yourself and the situations that have contributed to the way you deal with the world.

Sometimes psychotherapy is all you need to start feeling like yourself again. In other cases, a psychiatrist or physician may prescribe a medication to reduce your feelings of anxiety.

Conventional Medicines

In recent decades, benzodiazepines have replaced the more dangerous barbiturates that doctors used to prescribe for anxiety. Taken for short periods, benzodiazepines may be highly effective in alleviating your symptoms. But if you take them for too long, you may become addicted. In addition, many benzodiazepines cause adverse reactions. If you suffer from acute glaucoma (a sudden increase in pressure within the eye), for example, you should avoid several types of benzodiazepines, which could cause your symptoms to worsen. In addition, combining benzodiazepines with alcohol can be lethal.

Prescription for Kava

Capsules: Most herbalists say that 200 to 300 milligrams a day provides enough kava to produce therapeutic effects.

Commonly used to treat anxiety are the benzodiazepines lorazepam (Ativan), diazepam (Valium), alprazolam (Xanax), and clonazepam (Klonopin). All of the drugs are effective as short-term remedies. But they do come with side effects. Common side effects include dizziness, lightheadedness, clumsiness or unsteadiness, drowsiness, and slurred speech. They may also impair your ability to drive or operate machinery. Combining them with alcohol or other central nervous system depressants, such as antihistamines and certain pain medications, can intensify their effects and could lead to unconsciousness and even death. If you use them for long periods, you can develop a tolerance for them or become dependent on them. And, if you stop taking them suddenly, you may experience uncomfortable withdrawal symptoms, so you must be weaned from them gradually.

Another prescription option is buspirone (Buspar). But even buspirone can cause drowsiness, dizziness, headache, nausea, restlessness, nervousness, or unusual excitement. And if you have severe kidney or liver damage, you should not take buspirone.

If your anxiety is mild, you may want to consider a natural medicine called kava. The herb has been used for centuries to relieve anxiety, and it could help you as well. Read on, and then if you are interested, discuss kava with a physician experienced in both traditional and natural medicines.

What Is Kava?

You don't have to tackle traffic in Manhattan to experience stress. It's everywhere, even in the relative paradise of Polynesia. To deal with stress, and just to boost their spirits, many islanders drink a beverage produced from the kava kava root. Because of its reported ability to banish anxiety and induce feelings of bliss, kava has been revered for centuries in certain South Pacific islands and Hawaii.

The kava beverage produced in the islands imparts a mild numbing sensation to your tongue. This is followed by a sociable feeling of relaxation and a marked reduction in fatigue and anxiety.

In Europe and the United States, you aren't likely to ever encounter a cup of kava beverage. Instead, you can purchase capsules filled with powdered kava root. Kava has sedative, tonic, stimulant, diuretic, diaphoretic, and reportedly, aphrodisiac properties.

Just how kava works is unclear. Scientists have isolated several compounds from kava root. These so-called kava pyrones include kawain, dihydrokawain, methysticin, dihydromethysticin, yangonin, and dihydroyangonon.

Small amounts of kava produce euphoria. If you take larger amounts, you may feel extreme relaxation, lethargy, and a sense of sleepiness.

You may not appreciate kava's effects the first few times you try it. Some people need to become used to the herb before it kicks in.

In Germany, researchers conducted a double-blind study of 58 patients suffering from common anxiety syndromes. None of the patients was considered to be psychotic or to have a severe mental illness. Half of the patients received a placebo (a dummy pill). The other half took 100 milligrams of kava extract three times a day for four weeks. The researchers then administered several tests to assess patients' anxiety levels. These included the Hamilton Anxiety Scale, a 60-item Adjectives Check List self-assessment scale, and the Clinical Global Impression scale (CGI). After just one week, patients who took kava demonstrated a significant reduction in anxiety symptoms, compared with patients who took the placebo. What's more, the kava patients continued to improve throughout the 28-day study.

None of the patients who received kava complained of adverse reactions. Thus, researchers concluded, kava extract is "suitable for the general practitioner in treating states of anxiety, tension, and excitedness."

Arnold Fox, M.D., is one practitioner who advises his patients to try kava for anxiety problems. "If my patients are on Xanax [alprazolam] or Valium [diazepam], I'll try to switch them to kava," says Fox, "Taken as directed, kava is safe and often produces quite satisfactory results. Several studies back up its claims."

In one such study of kava's effects, 101 patients suffering from a variety of conditions—agoraphobia, specific phobia, generalized anxiety disorder, or adjustment disorder—were examined for 25 weeks at various mental health clinics. Half of the patients received a placebo. The other half took a special kava extract known as WS 1490.

Is Kava Safe?

Consumed in moderation, kava appears to be perfectly safe. However, overconsumption of the herb has caused a condition known in the Polynesian islands as Kawaism. Regular and prolonged use of kava may result in a yellow skin rash, which goes away after you stop using the herb. There are no ill effects from withdrawal.

Researchers then rated the subjects' anxiety levels with the Hamilton Anxiety Scale. Patients who had been taking kava for eight weeks scored far better than patients who took the placebo. The researchers reported that adverse reactions during the study were rare and distributed evenly among both groups. They concluded that kava is a good alternative to tricyclic antidepressants and benzodiazepines because of its "proven long-term efficacy and none of the tolerance problems associated with tricyclics and benzodiazepines."

German researchers also have found that kava produces deep muscle relaxation, modulates emotional processes, and promotes sleep as effectively as most tranquilizers.

The best news about kava is that it appears to be relatively free of side effects, at least in short-

Because kava may induce feelings of euphoria, excessive consumption may lead to abuse. Research shows, however, that kava is not physically addictive, and even in very high doses, kava has not caused death in laboratory animals.

Kava should be avoided during pregnancy and lactation. Care should also be taken before driving or operating machinery; be sure you know how kava affects you before attempting either.

term use. Unlike benzodiazepines, kava reduces anxiety but does not affect motor control, physical performance, or reaction time. Moderate doses of kava have even been shown in some clinical trials to improve cognitive performance, presumably by stabilizing emotional distress. Kava does not appear to interact adversely with alcohol, but for safety's sake, it is probably advisable to avoid combining the two.

In other tests, kava has calmed subjects but has had no adverse effects on electroencephalograph (EEG) readings of brain-wave activity.

No toxicity has been observed in people who took a moderate dose of 200 milligrams of kava a day for eight weeks. In doses greater than 8 ounces, or 30 capsules, per day for months, kava may cause a rash and skin discoloration.

If you suffer from a serious anxiety disorder, you may need pharmaceutical medicines as well as psychotherapy. But if your symptoms are mild, kava may help you out of a tough time. Discuss the herb with a doctor experienced in natural remedies. Then the two of you can decide whether kava may help you to reduce the anxiety that all of us find overwhelming from time to time.

INDEX

A

Acarbose, 226

Acetaminophen, 84, 103, 189–190, 206–207

Acupuncture, 182, 188, 190

Adenosine, 73

Adrenaline, 234

Alcohol, 10, 37, 44, 48, 50, 133, 233, 240, 242

Allicin, 68, 73

Allium sativum. See Garlic.

Alprazolam, 19, 243, 246

Alzheimer disease, 140–161
  and aluminum, 146
  causes, 146–147
  definition, 142–146
  ethnic component, 144–146, 148–149
  genetic component, 147–149
  incidence, 142
  symptoms, 142–146
  treatments for, 150–151

Amantadine, 85

Ambien, 35, 151

Amenorrhea, 186–188, 199

American Association of Naturopathic Physicians, 38

American Herbalist Guild, 30

American Holistic Medical Association, 40, 165, 185

Amitril, 37

Amitriptiline, 15, 24, 26, 37

Amyloid, 146

Anemia, 191

Angelica sinensis, 199

Anorexia, 188

Antacids, 124

Antibiotics, 85

Antibodies, 79

Antihistamines, 37–38, 84, 125

Antioxidants, 31, 34, 66, 67, 68, 151, 157, 223

Antispasmodics, 137

Anxiety, 7, 16, 17, 35, 44, 142, 155, 159, 167, 232–248
  defining, 233–235
  disorders, 235–241

Aphrodisiacs, 174

Arachidonic acid, 157

Aricept TM, 150

Aromatherapy, 182

Arthritis, 87, 96–115
  and exercise, 101–103
  causes, 99–100
  diagnosing, 100–101
  incidence of, 96, 97
  surgery for, 104–105
  symptoms, 97–99
  treatment, 101–105

Aspirin, 64, 70, 72, 84, 103, 104, 136, 189, 201, 206, 207

Association of Natural Medicine Pharmacists, 213

Asthma, 154

Atherosclerosis, 61, 66, 74–75

Aventyl, 15

Axid, 124

B

Bacteria, 78, 85, 87, 89, 90

Benign prostatic hyperplasia, 163–181

Bioflavonoids, 157

Bisabolol, 129

Black cohosh, 198–199, 199

Black haw bark, 189

Block, Eric, 65–66

Blood
  cells, 87, 89
  cholesterol, 55, 60–63
  circulation, 141
  clots, 57, 64, 66, 68, 72–73, 152, 153, 154, 157
  glucose, 221, 222, 223, 226–227, 227
  pressure. *See* Hypertension; Hypotension.
  "thinning," 64, 70, 72

Bloomfield, Harold, 21

BPH. *See* Benign prostatic hyperplasia.

Brain
  blood flow to, 13
  degeneration, 142
  function, 13, 154

Breggin, Peter, 18

Brewer's yeast, 228

Bronchitis, 175

Buckholz, Neil, 145–146

Buspar, 243

Buspirone, 243

C

Caffeine, 48, 206, 240

Calan, 210